MW01491893

THE COMPLETE

Pegan Diet

COOK BOOK

600 Delicious Fast and Easy Pegan Diet Recipe Combining the Best of Paleo and Vegan Diet for Life long Health

Cynthia L. Cantor

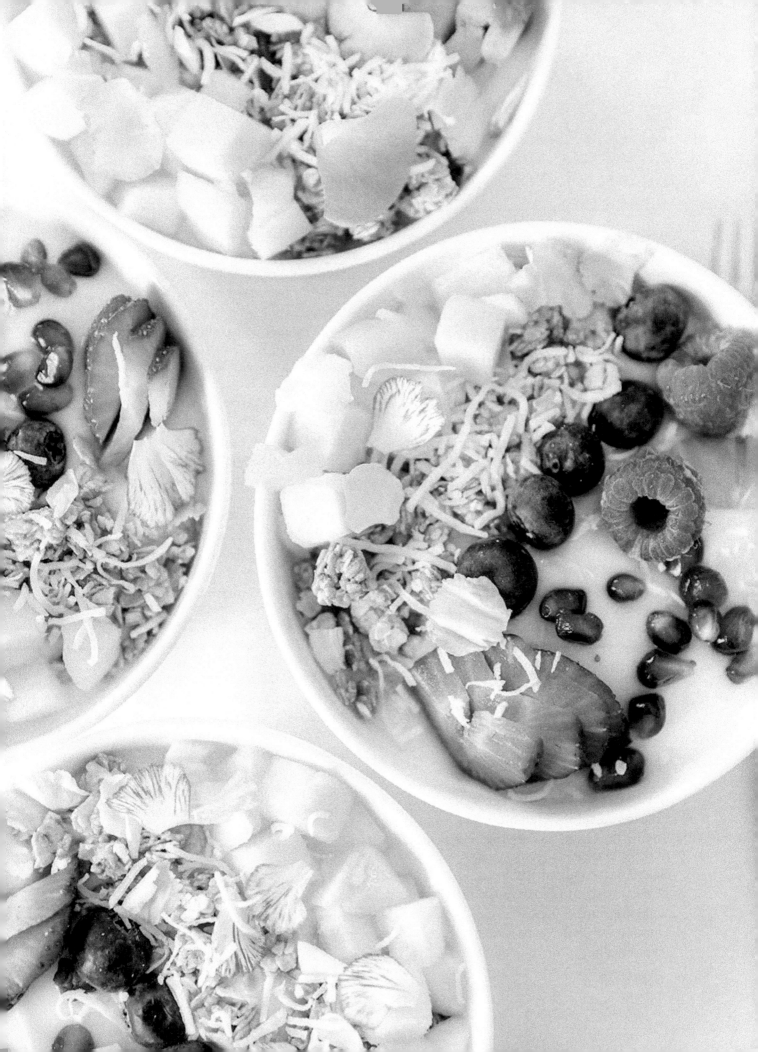

TABLE OF CONTENT

CHAPTER 5: DINNER RECIPES 47

CHAPTER 6: SMOOTHIES AND DRINKS............................... 65

CHAPTER 7: DESSERTS, APPETIZERS AND SNACKS 78

CHAPTER 8: SALADS, DRESSINGS, SOUPS AND STOCKS........................ 98

CHAPTER 9: SIDE DISHES 109

CHAPTER 10: SAUCES AND SPREADS 122

CHAPTER 11: MEAT & CHICKEN RECIPES..................................133

CHAPTER 12: PEGAN SEA FOOD RECIPES....................... 143

INTRODUCTION

The Pegan Diet is a combination of two very popular diets – the Paleo Diet and the Vegan Diet. The Paleo Diet is based on the eating habits of our Paleolithic-era ancestors and it includes only those foods which would have been available prior to the birth of agriculture. Vegan diet attempts to exclude all forms of animal exploitation and cruelty, whether for food, clothing or any other purpose. For these reasons, the vegan diet is devoid of all animal products, including meat, eggs and dairy. In fact, Pegan cooking offers you the best nutritional aspects of vegan and Paleo diets , the two dietary powerhouses, plus countless health benefits, such as improving your health, preventing disease, lowering inflammation, and boosting your energy levels.

Consequently, the two styles contradict each other in certain ways, but the main tenant that the Pegan diet follows is a focus on real, whole foods. The idea is to cut back on the processed stuff as followers of the diet eat vegetables, fruits, nuts, seeds, meat, fish, and eggs and avoid dairy, grains, legumes, sugar, and processed foods.

The Pegan diet discourages eating conventionally farmed meats or eggs. Instead, it places emphasis on grass-fed, pasture-raised sources of beef, pork, poultry, and whole eggs. It also encourages intake of fish — specifically those that tend to have low mercury content like sardines and wild salmon.

The Pegan diet restricts many nutrient-rich foods, partly because some people can't tolerate them. While it's true that some people are intolerant to lactose or gluten, or have trouble digesting the fiber in beans, that's not the case for most people. If someone follows the Pegan diet because they struggle with inflammation or digestive health, it will help discovering the root cause of their health problems as well.

CHAPTER 1 UNDERSTANDING PEGAN DIET

WHAT IS PEGAN DIET?

It's the Blending of Vegan and Paleo Diets into One Healthy Plan. The concept of Pegan Diet originated in the year 2016 with Dr. Mark Hyman, the director of The Ultra Wellness Center and a world-renowned leader in Functional Medicine, as a way to promote proper eating for overall well-being. Dr. Mark Hyman is the leading voice for Functional Medicine in America and has devoted his life to understanding how lifestyle choices can change our genes. In his book, he has deliberated about all the benefits of Pegan Diet, thus you can thank him for this great concept.

Peganizing diet means to include the aspects of both vegetarian and Paleo diets in your daily routine. The basic idea is to eliminate all processed foods from the daily routine and introduce healthier options like vegetables, fruits, nuts, seeds, eggs etc. and Include cereals like amaranth, buckwheat or quinoa in case you are allergic to gluten or if you have a gluten intolerance. In order to get a clear understanding, you should know what vegan diet is and what Paleo diet is as well.

ADDING VEGAN AND PALEO DIET FOR PEGAN DIET

What is Vegan Diet?

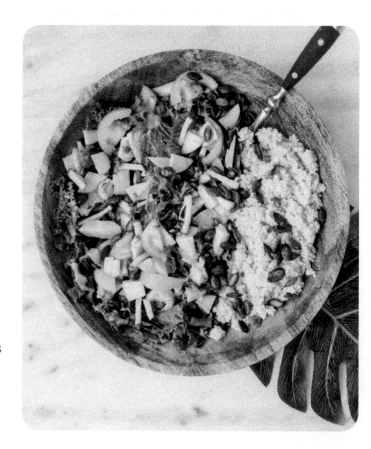

The vegan diet avoids the consumption of all animal-derived products, including dairy and eggs. Vegan, by definition, is a word used to explain a complete lifestyle, one that is lived in a manner that avoids as much harm to sentient beings as possible. Ethical vegans not only shun all animal products in food; they also eliminate use of animal-sourced items in their overall day-to-day lives. Products deriving from animals or exploiting creatures in some manner, including leather, wool, silk, pearls, and beeswax, do not fit into the vegan lifestyle.

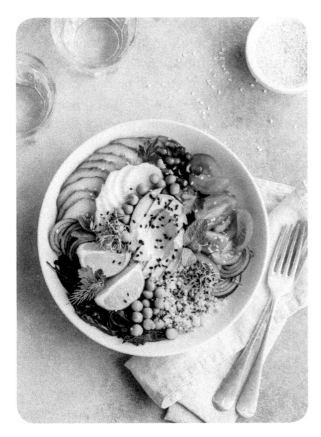

Ethical vegans have long touted the health benefits received from eating only plant-based foods. A well-planned vegan diet is high in fiber and low in saturated fat, and incorporates above-average consumption of fruits and vegetables. Additionally, cholesterol is not consumed in any amount.

Cholesterol, a sterol that is produced by the liver and occurs in all cells of the body, is found in all animal products. Although the waxy substance is essential for life, the body produces all it needs to function properly. Consuming too much cholesterol can be dangerous, as it leads to plaque formation between the layers of the artery walls, making the heart work harder to circulate blood. Studies show that vegans have a lower risk of some of today's biggest health issues, including type 2 diabetes, cardiovascular disease, obesity, and some forms of cancer, possibly due to the absence of cholesterol in the diet.

What Are the Disadvantages of the Vegan Diet?

Adopting a vegan diet means cutting out all animal products and achieving protein requirements through grains and legumes. Because of this, the vegan diet can be lacking in certain vital nutrients such as protein, calcium, B12, folate, and omega-3 fatty acids. The Pegan diet allows organic, sustainably raised animal products, preventing the risk of nutrition deficiencies.

On the vegan diet, many people eat forms of refined carbohydrates, including white bread, white pasta, and white sugar. Certain inflammatory foods are also allowed on the vegan diet—including artificial sweeteners, refined oils, and processed foods—since they do not come from animals. These inflammatory foods are highly discouraged on the Pegan diet, as they are associated with obesity and disease.

What is Paleo Diet?

The Paleo diet celebrates the foods that were consumed during the Palaeolithic era, also called the Old Stone Age—a time period that extended from the beginning of human existence (2.5 million years ago) until approximately 12,000 B.C.E. Palaeolithic people were hunter-gatherers whose diet consisted only of items found in nature—meats, poultry, fish, insects, eggs, leafy greens, fruits, berries, nuts, and seeds. Today's Paleo embraces the same pre-agricultural diet as that of his ancient ancestors. The Paleo diet is filled with foods that would have been hunted and gathered by cavemen. Of course, in today's modern society, those consuming a Paleo diet need not head to the forest, fields, and streams to find their food. It's simply a matter of understanding the dos and don'ts of primitive foods.

The Paleo diet has become increasingly popular with people looking to live a healthier lifestyle. Because processed foods and refined sugars are shunned and dairy and carbs are eliminated, the diet is used to develop a lean yet muscular body composition. Additionally, it is believed that the Paleo lifestyle has many health benefits, including increased energy levels and reduced risk of diseases such as diabetes, heart disease, obesity, and cancer.

What Are the Disadvantages of the Paleo Diet?

Because of its heavy emphasis on animal protein, the Paleo diet can be difficult for a vegetarian or vegan to follow. The Paleo diet also gives some an excuse to pile their plates with meat while conveniently forgetting about the vegetables. In addition, the elimination of grains, potatoes, and beans limits the variety of fiber-containing foods allowed on this diet. This may lead to a decreased intake of fiber, which you need for gut health.

The Paleo diet is also fairly restrictive and can be difficult to follow long-term, especially while traveling or dining out. The Pegan diet includes all of the Paleo-approved foods plus more, including potatoes, gluten-free grains, beans, peas, and unprocessed forms of soy. This allows for more variety and flexibility, making the Pegan diet more suitable for a long-term lifestyle change.

The Best of 2 Worlds: Vegan+Pegan=The Pegan Diet

To optimize the health benefits of the vegan diet and Paleo diets, the Pegan diet emphasizes whole, real foods that are unprocessed. The Pegan diet was created by Mark Hyman, MD. Foods that come from a box are not Pegan friendly. In fact, many of the foods you will purchase won't even have a nutrition label. You will likely find yourself shopping the perimeter of the grocery store.

The Pegan diet advocates choosing locally sourced, organic, and sustainably raised foods. During your Pegan adventure, you may decide to start exploring local farmers' markets or shopping at grocery stores with larger organic produce sections. This is a lifestyle change that will intensify your appreciation of healthy foods and force you outside your comfort zone.

The Pegan diet promotes optimal health by reducing inflammation and balancing blood sugar. It is believed that the Pegan lifestyle has many health benefits, including weight loss, increased energy levels, and reduced risk of diseases such as diabetes, heart disease, obesity, and cancer.

What do a Pegan Eat?

The Pegan diet includes both plant-based foods and animal products; however the diet emphasizes filling the majority of your plate with vegetables. Fruits and no starchy vegetables should comprise 75 percent of your diet. With a focus on reducing inflammation, the Pegan diet is rich in healthy fats such as fish, eggs, olive oil, avocado, nuts (excluding peanuts), and seeds. The diet also incorporates gluten-free grains such as quinoa, rice, oats, and millet which are a great source of fiber. Grain intake should not exceed more than 1/2 cup per meal to help regulate blood sugar levels.

Beans and lentils offer a great source of vegetarian protein. Other foods such as potatoes and goat and sheep products are encouraged in moderation. For a complete food list, see Appendix: Pegan "Yes" Foods. Pro-inflammatory foods such as gluten, refined sugar, processed soy, refined oils, food additives, and dairy products are strongly discouraged

Where Do Pegans Get Protein?

Pegans can eat both animal and plant proteins. If a vegetarian wanted to follow the Pegan diet, it would be very doable! Vegetarian sources of protein include black beans, pinto beans, lentils, edamame, chickpeas, quinoa, nuts, and seeds. Many individuals overeat protein while under eating fresh fruits and vegetables. The Pegan diet prevents this by setting appropriate meal guidelines. Animal protein such as steak, chicken, pork, and fish should be limited to a palm-sized serving, approximately 3 to 6 ounces per meal. Beans and lentil intake should not exceed more than 1 cup per day

Pegan Sweeteners

The Pegan diet recommends sweeteners to be used sparingly. Sweeteners with a low glycaemic load (GL) are preferred, including honey, maple syrup, and coconut sugar.

The term glycemic load refers to a measurement used to determine how much a consumed food will raise the body's blood glucose. GL is calculated by multiplying the food's glycaemic index (GI) number by the carbohydrates in a serving. Pegans choose to consume items with low glycaemic loads because the lower value has less impact on the body's blood sugar levels. By keeping the levels more consistent and avoiding sharp raises, a low-glycaemic diet helps stabilize the body's weight and, in turn, prevents obesity-related diseases. Low GI foods are also connected to improved moods and increased energy.

The Part-Time Pegan

When studied separately, both the vegan diet and the Paleo diet have been shown to reduce the chances of certain diseases. No doubt, when combined, the resulting Pegan diet has extensive health benefits. Even so, it may be difficult to follow a strict Pegan diet on a full-time basis. With that in mind, there is no harm in choosing one diet as your main lifestyle and incorporating meals that meet the requirements of both. Think of it as a Pegan challenge of sorts. Start with at least one meal a day that includes foods that adhere to the diet.

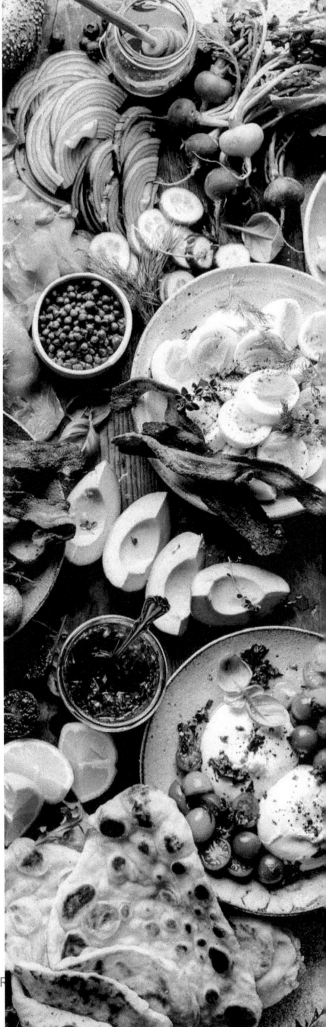

THE GUIDELINES FOR THE PEGAN DIET

The Pegan diet focuses strongly on whole foods, or foods that have undergone little to no processing before they make it to your plate.

1. Eat lots of plants

The primary food group for the Pegan diet is vegetables and fruit — these should comprise 75% of your total intake. Low-glycaemic fruits and vegetables, such as berries and non-starchy vegetables should be emphasized in order to minimize your blood sugar response. Small amounts of starchy vegetables and sugary fruits may be allowed for those who have already achieved healthy blood sugar control prior to starting the diet.

2. Choose responsibly sourced protein

Although the Pegan diet primarily emphasizes plant foods, adequate protein intake from animal sources is still encouraged. Bear in mind that because 75% of the diet is made up of vegetables and fruit, less than 25% remains for animal-based proteins. As such, you'll have a much lower meat intake than you would on a typical Paleo diet — but still more than on any vegan diet.

The Pegan diet discourages eating conventionally farmed meats or eggs. Instead, it places emphasis on grass-fed, pasture-raised sources of beef, pork, poultry, and whole eggs. It also encourages intake of fish — specifically those that tend to have low mercury content like sardines and wild salmon.

3. Stick to minimally processed fats

On this diet, you should eat healthy fats from specific sources, such as:

- **Nuts:** Except peanuts
- **Seeds:** Except processed seed oils
- **Avocado and olives:** Cold-pressed olive and avocado oil may also be used
- **Coconut:** Unrefined coconut oil is permitted
- **Omega-3s:** Especially those from low-mercury fish or algae

Grass-fed, pasture-raised meats and whole eggs also contribute to the fat content of the Pegan diet.

4. Some whole grains and legumes may be consumed

Although most grains and legumes are discouraged on the Pegan diet due to their potential to influence blood sugar, some gluten-free whole grains and legumes are permitted in limited quantities. Grain intake should not exceed more than a 1/2 cup (125 grams) per meal, while legume intake should not exceed 1 cup (75 grams) per day.

Here are some grains and legumes that you may eat:

- **Grains:** Black rice, quinoa, amaranth millet, teff, oats
- **Legumes:** Lentils, chickpeas, black beans, pinto beans

However, you should further restrict these foods if you have diabetes or another condition that contributes to poor blood sugar control

FOODS TO INCLUDE IN PEGAN DIET

FRUITS AND VEGETABLES

- Apples, red
- Artichoke hearts, water packed
- Avocados
- Baby spinach
- Basil, fresh
- Beets
- Bell peppers, green, red, yellow, or orange
- Blackberries
- Bok choy
- Cabbage, red or Napa
- Carrots
- Celery
- Chard, Swiss or rainbow
- Chives, fresh
- Cilantro, fresh
- Collard greens
- Cucumber
- Eggplant
- Frozen blueberries
- Garlic
- Ginger
- Green beans
- Kale
- Lemons
- Lettuce, Boston, Bib, red leaf, or romaine
- Limes
- Mushrooms
- Olives
- Onions, yellow or red
- Oregano, fresh
- Parsley, flat-leaf
- Peppers, jalapeño or Serrano
- Raspberries
- Rosemary, fresh
- Scallions
- Shallots
- Squash, butternut, spaghetti, acorn, yellow, or summer
- Strawberries
- Sweet potatoes
- Tomatillos
- Tomatoes, fresh
- Zucchini

MEAT AND POULTRY

- Beef, grass-fed
- Bison, grass-fed
- Butter, grass-fed
- Chicken, pastured or organic, no antibiotics
- Eggs, pastured or organic
- Game, elk or venison
- Lamb, pastured, grass-fed
- Pork, pastured or crate-free
- Turkey, pastured

SEA FOOD

- Arctic char, wild
- Clams, canned or fresh
- Cod
- Crab, canned or fresh
- Flounder
- Herring, wild-caught
- Lobster
- Mackerel, Atlantic or Pacific
- Mussels
- Oysters
- Salmon, wild-caught, fresh or canned
- Sardines, fresh or canned
- Scallops
- Shrimp
- Snapper
- Tilapia
- Trout
- Tuna, line-caught, albacore, fresh or canned

NUTS AND SEEDS

- Almond butter, raw or dry-roasted, unsalted
- Almonds, raw
- Brazil nuts, raw
- Cashew butter, roasted, unsalted
- Cashews, raw
- Chia seeds
- Flaxseeds
- Hazelnuts, raw or dry-roasted, unsalted
- Macadamia nuts, raw or dry-roasted, unsalted
- Pecans, raw, unsalted

- Pine nuts, from Italian sources only
- Pistachios, raw or dry-roasted, unsalted
- Pumpkin seeds (pepitas), raw or dry-roasted, unsalted
- Sesame seeds, toasted
- Walnuts, whole or chopped, raw, unsalted*

PANTRY ITEMS

- Avocado oil
- Broth or stock, unsalted
- Cacao powder, raw
- Coconut flakes, unsweetened
- Coconut oil
- Dates, Medjool
- Honey, raw, from sustainable sources (see Choosing the Right Honey)
- Hot sauce, no additives
- Maple syrup, no additives

- Miso
- Mustard, Dijon
- Nori sheets
- Nutritional yeast
- Olive oil, extra-virgin, cold-pressed
- Salsa, no sugar or additives
- Sesame oil
- Soy sauce, gluten-free, tamari, or coconut amino
- Sriracha
- Tempeh
- Tofu, sprouted
- Tomatoes, no sugar or salt added, crushed, chopped, or whole, boxed
- Vanilla, extra pure, no alcohol
- Vinegars, balsamic, red wine, cider, sherry, rice, coconut
- Wasabi paste

SPICES

- Bay leaves
- Black pepper or peppercorns
- Cayenne pepper
- Chilli powder
- Cinnamon, ground
- Cumin, ground
- Curry powder
- Garlic powder
- Nutmeg, whole
- Onion powder
- Oregano, dried
- Paprika, hot, sweet, or smoked
- Red pepper flakes
- Thyme, dried
- Turmeric
- Salt (sea salt and pink salt ; kosher salt is also good)

MUST AVOID FOODS IN PEGAN DIET

The Pegan diet is more flexible than a Paleo or vegan diet because it allows occasional intake of almost any food. Several foods and food groups are strongly discouraged. Some of these foods are known to be unhealthy, while others may be considered very healthy — depending on whom you ask.

These foods are typically avoided on the Pegan diet:

- **Dairy:** Cow's milk, yogurt, and cheese are strongly discouraged. However, foods made from sheep or goat milk are permitted in limited quantities. Sometimes grass-fed butter is allowed, too.

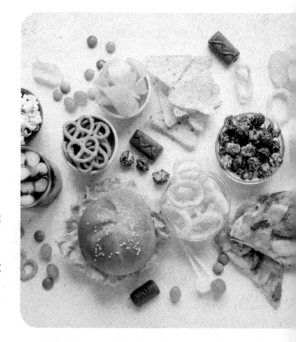

- **Gluten:** All gluten-containing grains are strongly discouraged.

- **Gluten-free grains:** Even grains that don't contain gluten are discouraged. Small amounts of gluten-free whole grains may be permitted occasionally.

- **Legumes:** Most legumes are discouraged due to their potential to increase blood sugar. Low-starch legumes, such as lentils may be permitted.

- **Sugar:** Any form of added sugar, refined or not, is usually avoided. It may be used occasionally — but very sparingly.

- **Refined oils:** Refined or highly processed oils, such as canola, soybean, sunflower, and corn oil, are almost always avoided.

- **Food additives:** Artificial colourings, flavourings, preservatives, and other additives are avoided.

Most of these foods are forbidden due to their perceived impact on blood sugar and/ or inflammation in your body.

OTHER RULES ON THE PEGAN DIET

- Limit starchy veggies such as potatoes or winter squash (no more than ½ cup per day), and stick to lower-sugar fruits such as berries and kiwi. Beans should be eaten sparingly (less than 1 cup per day.)

- Non-gluten-containing whole grains (teff, black rice, quinoa, and amaranth) may be eaten sparingly (½ cup per meal.)

- Sugar in the form of maple syrup or honey may be had as an occasional treat.

- Occasional grass-fed, organic cow's milk dairy products such as ghee or kefir may be eaten, if they do not cause discomfort; sheep's milk and goat's milk products may also be enjoyed.

- Foods should be minimally processed and as close to their whole-food form as possible.

- While there's no specific mention of alcohol, it is generally forbidden on the Paleo diet.

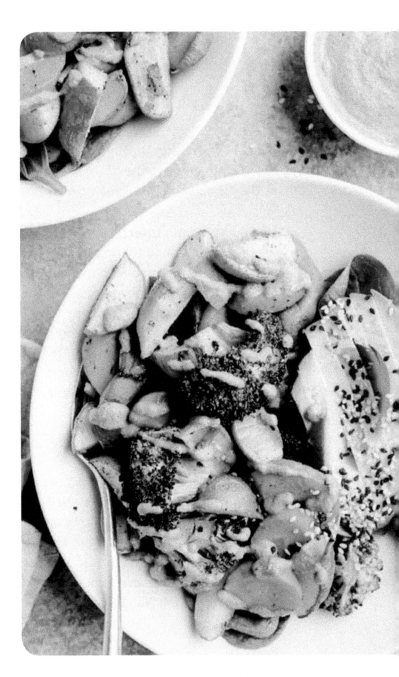

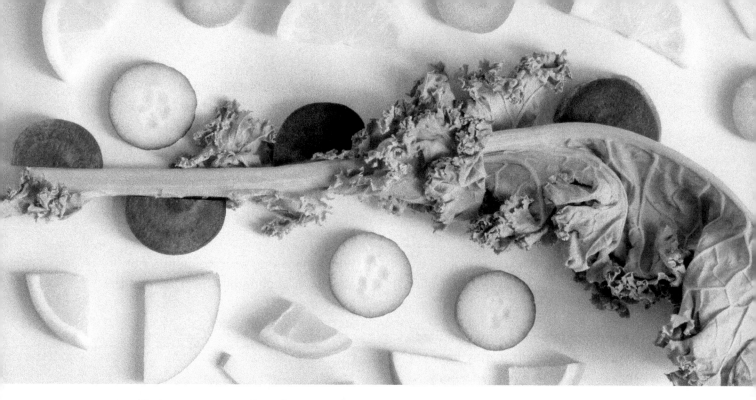

13 PILLARS OF THE PEGAN DIET

The Pegan Diet Creator, Dr. Mark Hyman, MD, says a Pegan diet combines principles of Paleo and vegan diets and it is the best way to eat. Here are the 13 pillars of the Pegan diet. Let's look at the 13 pillars of the Pegan diet.

1. **Stay away from sugar.** That means a diet low in anything that causes a spike in our insulin production — sugar, flour, and refined carbohydrates. Think of sugar in all its various forms as an occasional treat, that is, something we eat occasionally and sparingly. It is as a recreational drug. You use it for fun occasionally, but it is not a dietary staple.

2. **Eat mostly plants.** More than half your plate should be covered with veggies. The deeper the color, the better. The more variety, the healthier. Stick with mostly no starchy veggies. Winter squashes and sweet potatoes are fine in moderation (1/2 cup a day). Not a ton of potatoes! French fries don't count even though they are the No. 1 vegetable in America.

3. **Easy on fruits.** Stick with berries, kiwis, and watermelon, and watch the grapes, melons, and so on. Think of dried fruit as candy and keep it to a minimum.

4. **Stay away from pesticides, antibiotics, hormones, and GMO foods.** Also, no chemicals, additives, preservatives, dyes, artificial sweeteners, or other junk ingredients. If you don't have that ingredient in your kitchen for cooking, you shouldn't eat it.

5. **Eat foods containing healthy fats.** I'm talking about omega-3 fatty acids and other good fats like those we find in nuts, seeds, olive oil, and avocados. And yes, we can even eat saturated fat from fish, whole eggs, and grass-fed or sustainably raised meat, grass-fed butter or ghee, and organic virgin coconut oil or coconut butter.

6. **Stay away from most vegetable, nut, and seed oils,** such as canola, sunflower, corn, grape seed, and especially soybean oil, which now accounts for about 10 percent of our calories. Small amounts of expeller or cold-pressed nut and seed oils like sesame, macadamia, and walnut oils are fine to use as condiments or for flavoring. Avocado oil is great for higher-temperature cooking.

7. **Avoid or limit dairy.** Dairy doesn't work for most people, so avoid it, except for the occasional yogurt, kefir, grass fed butter, ghee, and even cheese if it doesn't cause any problems for you. Try goat or sheep products instead of cow dairy. And always go organic and grass-fed.

8. **Think of meat and animal products** as condiments Vegetables should take center stage, and meat should be the side dish. Servings should be 4 to 6 ounces, tops, per meal. I often make three or four vegetable side dishes.

9. **Eat sustainably raised or harvested low-mercury fish.** If you are eating fish, you should choose low-mercury and low-toxin varieties such as sardines, herring, anchovies, and wild-caught salmon (all of which have high omega-3 and low mercury levels). And they should be sustainably harvested or farmed.

10. **Avoid gluten.** Most gluten comes from "Franken wheat," so look for heirloom varieties of wheat like einkorn. Eat wheat only if you are not gluten-sensitive and, even then, only occasionally. Since gluten damages the gut even in no gluten-sensitive people who show no symptoms.

11. **Eat gluten-free whole grains sparingly.** They still raise blood sugar and can trigger autoimmunity. All grains can increase your blood sugar. Stick with small portions (1/2 cup per meal) of low-glycaemic grains like black rice, quinoa, teff, buckwheat, or amaranth. For type 2 diabetics and those with autoimmune disease or digestive disorders, a grain- and bean-free diet may be key to treating and even reversing your illness.

12. **Eat beans only once in a while.** Lentils are best. Stay away from big starchy beans. Beans can be a great source of fiber, protein, and minerals. But they cause digestive problems for some, and the lectins and phytates they contain may impair mineral absorption. If you are diabetic, a high-bean diet can trigger spikes in your blood sugar. Again, moderate amounts (up to 1 cup a day) are OK.

13. **Get tested to personalize your approach.** What works for one person may not work for another. This is called bio-individuality and it is why he recommends that everyone eventually work with a functionally trained nutritionist to personalize his or her diet even further with the right tests.

CHAPTER 2 THE PEGAN DIET ACTION PLAN

PANTRY STOCK FOR THE 21-DAY PEGAN MEAL PLAN

This is not a quick fix that you follow for 21 days and then quit. After you reset your body, eat this way every single day. It is inclusive, not exclusive, and based on sound nutritional science. Stock up in your pantry with the below ingredients so that you can easily prepare delicious and healthy Pegan Meals.

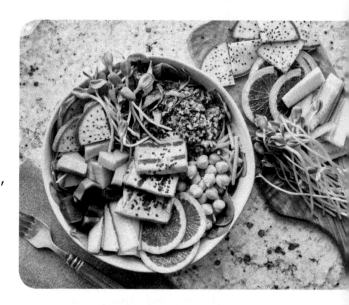

Pegan Pantry Stock: Oils/Vinegars/Sauces
Tamari: a great gluten-free soy sauce alternative made of fermented soy beans. Works well if sauces, dips, stir-fries, and dressings.
Coconut Amino: a soy-free soy sauce alternative, with a lighter flavour than tamari. Works well if sauces, dips, stir-fries, and dressings.
Olive Oil: For low-heat cooking, dressings, marinades, and drizzling.
Avocado Oil: For higher heat cooking and roasting.
Grass-Fed Ghee: Ghee is a by-product of butter, made by slowly simmering butter then straining off the milk solids.
Unfiltered Apple Cider Vinegar: It is used for marinades, dressings, and for general health maintenance or when we are sick
Primal Kitchen Dressings: Usually for Greek and lemon Turmeric dressing

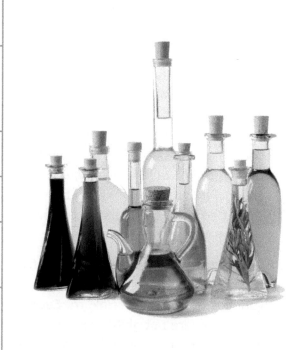

Pegan Pantry: Herbs & Spices

Turmeric: A bright yellow aromatic powder with powerful anti-inflammatory properties obtained from a plant of the ginger family. Sprinkle it in meals especially curries and Asian dishes, but also as a substitute for fresh turmeric.

Cumin: Use it in Mexican and Asian dishes mostly. It's the aromatic seeds of a plant of the parsley family, usually ground.

Garlic Granules: Granules are dehydrated finely minced garlic that tends to have a stronger taste than garlic powder. Sprinkle these on veggies before roasting.

Spice Blends: For taco spice blend, Italian blend, and Greek blend on hand for easing seasoning.

Tea: For green tea and Ginger Turmeric tea Dandelion Root tea

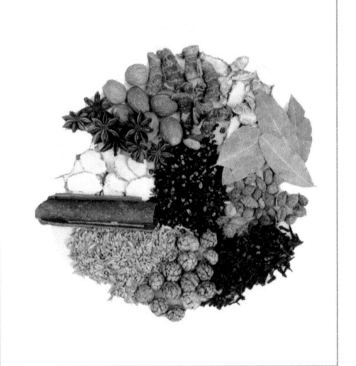

Pegan Pantry: Dry Goods

Almond Flour: Used in Paleo baking.

Coconut Flour: Used in Paleo baking.

Arrowroot Powder: a white, flavourless powder used to thicken sauces and soups, but also used in a lot of gluten-free baking and cooking,

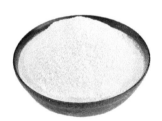

Pegan Pantry: Nuts/Seeds/Grains

Dates: For sweetening smoothies, dressings, baked goods, etc.

Cashews: Makes delicious, creamy, dairy-free sauces, thickens soups, delicious on their own.

Chia Seeds: For chia puddings for breakfast, smoothies, to sprinkle on top of yogurt, peanut butter banana toast etc.

Ground Flaxseed: For adding to smoothies and Paleo baked goods.

Almond Butter: For smoothies, for toast, for eating off a spoon.

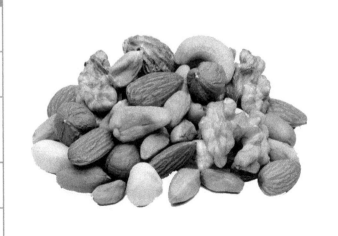

Brazil Nuts: Rich in selenium, I eat one a day to help with hormones and keep a strong immune system.	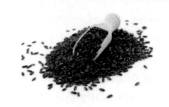
Quinoa	
Black Rice	

Pegan Pantry: Canned and Jarred Goods	
Organic Canned Chicken: To add a quick protein to lunch wraps.	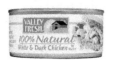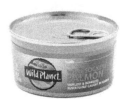
Wild Caught Canned Salmon: Use this to make these salmon burgers (sub panko)	
Olives: For snacking like black olives, kalamata olives, and castelvetrano (so buttery!)	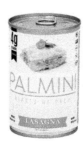
Coconut Milk: a delicious base to a plethora of yummy sauces, and can also be blended into coffee or smoothies.	
Palmini: its 100% hearts of palm, cut into linguine "noodles." No fillers or weird ingredients, just hearts of palm. It has a great texture and it's so easy to just drain and heat.	

4 WEEK MEAL PLAN WITH MOTIVATIONAL QUOTES

Day	Breakfast	Lunch	Dinner	Snack/Dessert	Motivational Quotes
1	Spicy Egg pepper Zoodles with Avocado	Easy Veggie Turkey Mix	Beef Sliced with Lemony Arugula	Simple Vegan Brownies	Life changes very quickly, in a very positive way, if you let it.
2	Spicy garlicky vegan Frittata	Lemony Quinoa Salad with Peppery Tuna	Grilled Salmon & cucumber zucchini Salad	Homemade Olive Smoothie	Food can be both enjoyable and nourishing.
3	Black pepper spiced Avocado with Baked Eggs	Spicy and Garlicky Sweet Potato with Spinach	Homemade Chicken Carrot Soup	Vanilla flavoured Fresh Blueberry pie	I am a better person when I have less on my plate

4	Best Pumpkin cake ever	Classic Five Fruit Salad	Instant Parmesan Halibut	Salty Brown Apple	Let food be thy medicine and medicine be thy food.
5	Garlic roasted Brussels sprouts with pepper	Paleo Cauliflower Gnocchi with spinach	Fresh Vegetables and Beef Soup	Big Fat Dark Chocolate Cookies	If I don't eat junk, I don't gain weight.
6	Baked Spicy pepper Muffins	Sweet Potato Mango Soup topped with Vinaigrette	Spicy Chicken with Fresh Cilantro	Easy Papaya Mango Avocado Bowl	Keep an open mind and a closed refrigerator.
7	Peppery Eggs with Lemon Hollandaise Sauce	Baked Chicken Tenders with Toasted Coconut	Super Tasty Peppery Beef with Tomato	Epic Eggplant Puree recipe	Start where you are. Use what you have. Do what you can.
8	Strawberry banana protein Smoothie	Cauli-Muffins with Italian seasoning	Garlic Lamb with Kidney Beans	Hot and Spicy Zucchini Sticks	The hard days are what make you stronger.
9	Strawberry banana protein Smoothie	Crispy Chicken with Sweet Potato & Broccoli Tots	Sweet and Spicy Orange Chicken	Super Creamy Sesame Smoothie with Paprika	My body is less judgmental of my diet than my mind is.
10	Maple Walnut Almond Granola	Coconut Pork chops with Cinnamon sweet potato	Homemade Pineapple grilled Chicken	Mango Tangerines and Cilantro Bowl	Let food be thy medicine and medicine be thy food.
11	Thyme flavoured baked Eggs with Asparagus and Tomatoes	Creamy Peppery Cauliflower with Parsley	Hot & Spicy Pineapple Coconut Chicken	Chef's favourite Classic Avocado salad	New meal; fresh start.
12	Sugar free Blueberry Banana Pancakes	Baked vegetables with Lemon Tahini Sauce	Nutty Fruity Chicken with Zucchini Noodles	Dark Chocolate Nut Clusters	You didn't gain all your weight in one day; you won't lose it in one day. Be patient with yourself.
13	Almond and carrot Superhero Muffins	Scallion Mushroom Zoodles Salad with Basil	Rosemary Pepper Chicken with Broccoli Florets	Olive Oil Roasted Almonds	Ability is what you're capable of doing. Motivation determines what you do. Attitude determines how well you do it.

14	Very veggie Cauliflower Potato Hash	Simple Belgian endive Egg with Cheese and Onion	Apple Glazed Roasted Turkey Breast	Perfectly Roasted Parsnip Chips	I always believed if you take care of your body it will take care of you.
15	Oven Baked Asparagus with Eggs and Tomatoes	Carrot and Onion Scrambled Egg	Sweet and spicy Arrowroot Flank St	Pecan and Walnut Holiday Nut Mix	Looking after my health today gives me a better hope for tomorrow.
16	Healthy Roasted Nuts and seeds	Cheesy red Onions With sautéed Kale	Beef Cauliflower stir fry with Cilantro leaves	Sweet and Spicy Cashew Almond Mix	You may be disappointed if you fail, but you are doomed if you don't try.
17	Healthy Coconut Granola	Cheesy Ham and Onion scrambled Egg	Beef Bowl with Plum Tomato and Lentils	Ghee roasted Almond Pecan Mix	Fitness is like marriage; you can't cheat on it and expect it to work.
18	Breakfast Cranberry and Almond porridge	Perfect Broccoli scrambled eggs	Fresh Peas and Ground Beef with Almonds	Lemony Dates with Hazelnuts	Exercise should be regarded as a tribute to the heart.
19	Best Pumpkin cake ever	Easy No Mayo Apple Cabbage Slaw	Classic Beef-Zucchini Stuffed Peppers	Grandma's Special Caramel-Nuts Mix	If it doesn't challenge you, it doesn't change you.
20	Poached Apple and Pears with Cinnamon	Celery -Broccoli Macaroni Salad	Creamy Mushroom Pepper curry soup	Almond Strawberry Pumpkin Salad	It's going to be a journey. It's not a sprint to get in shape.
21	Lemony Avocado Salman Wraps	Easy Tomato Basil and Red Onion Salad	Homemade Lemon and Garlic Salmon	Mulberry-Pistachio Salad	Just believe in yourself. Even if you don't, pretend that you do and, at some point, you will.
22	Cheesy Toasted Golden Bagel with Tomato	Spicy Pasta with Mackerel and Breadcrumbs	One Pot Mustard Chicken with Bacon and Onions	Homemade-Coconut Oil Baked Seeds Mix	Nobody is perfect, so get over the fear of being or doing everything perfectly. Besides, perfect is boring.
23	Homemade Apple Cinnamon Oat Meal	Tasty Asparagus Noodles with Soy sauce	Ground Turkey with fresh Spinach and Tomato	Salty Brown Apple	The secret of change is to focus all of your energy not on fighting the old, but on building the new.

24	Chicken Cucumber Tomato Salad	Instant Tasty Cheesy Pizza with Tomato sauce	Baked Lemon Haddock	Chilled Coconut Banana Dessert	You get what you focus on, so focus on what you want.
25	Salmon Egg Sandwich with Avocado	Super Tasty Buttermilk Chicken Salad	Homemade White pepper Tomato Pasta	Vanilla flavoured Berry Mix Bowl	Yes, I can.
26	Perfect hard boiled Eggs for Two	Amazing Olive Pasta and Tomato Salad	Curried Shrimp and Cauliflower with Cilantro	Chocolate flavoured Almond Ball	Don't stop until you're proud.
27	Instant Moist Eggs with scallion greens	Mushroom Coconut Cream Soup	Grandma's Special Spinach Artichokes Stuff	Healthy Date Coconut Flake Cookies	A little progress each day adds up to big results.
28	Butter Egg omelette with Pepper	Super Tasty Buttermilk Chicken Salad	Quinoa with Peppery Oyster Mushrooms	Cinnamon Nutty Fruity Dessert	It has to be hard so you'll never ever forget

WHAT TO DO AFTER 28 DAYS

The Pegan diet is an important diet plan as it is effective for people suffering from type 2 diabetes and risk of cardiovascular diseases. Studies show that it takes 21 days to develop a habit and this is also true if you want to get used to healthy eating style. This 'food as medicine' way of eating is designed to help us live longer, lower inflammation and slow climate change.

You're shown how to prepare food in the Pegan Diet way, with advice on how to cook vegetables to make them tasty and the importance of neither overdoing nor undercooking your protein. The recipes are divided up into breakfast, lunch, dinner, soups and salads, sides, snacks and desserts.

By the end of 21 days, you will be able to observe significant differences in your body. But this does not mean that you should stop and revert to your usual eating habits. The thing is that your condition can easily come back, especially if you are not too careful about the things that you eat. If you're interested in veganism, but don't want to go completely meat-free, this could offer a viable alternative provided that the guidelines are adapted to suit your particular needs and lifestyle. It is pretty tricky though and so won't be for everyone, with its stance on grains sure to ruffle a few feathers in light of new findings. That is said though, because some gluten-free grains are included, it is less restrictive than a traditional Paleo diet.

CHAPTER 3: BREAKFAST RECIPES

Spicy Egg pepper Zoodles with Avocado

Prep time: 15 minutes | Cook time: 10 minutes | Serves 2

Non-stick spray
3 zucchinis, spiral zed into noodles
2 tablespoons extra-virgin olive oil
Kosher salt and freshly ground black pepper

4 large eggs
Red-pepper flakes, for garnishing
Fresh basil, for garnishing
2 avocados, halved and thinly sliced

1. Preheat the oven to 350°F.
2. Grease a baking sheet lightly with -stick spray.
3. Toss the zucchini noodles and olive oil to combine in a large bowl. Season it with salt and pepper. Divide into 4 even portions, transfer to the baking sheet and shape each into a nest.
4. Gently crack an egg into the Centre of each nest.
5. Bake until the eggs are set, 9 to 11 minutes. Season with salt and pepper; garnish with red-pepper flakes and basil.
6. Serve alongside the avocado slices.

Per Serving

Calorie 633| Fats 53g| Carbs 27g| Protein 20g

Strawberry banana protein Smoothie

Prep time: 5 minutes | Cook time: 1 minute | Serves 2

2 cups frozen strawberries
1 Teaspoon vanilla extract
1 cup coconut milk

1 frozen banana sliced
1 scoop collagen protein powder

1. Add all ingredients to a high-speed blender and blend until smooth.

Per Serving

Calorie 376 | Fats 24g| Carbs 27g| Protein 8g

Watercress Tomato Juice

Prep time: 20 minutes | Cook time: 15 minutes | Serves 5

1 cup chopped watercress
2 large tomatoes
2 medium stalks celery
1/2 large lemon,

peeled
1 tablespoon horseradish
1/2 teaspoon cayenne pepper
1 cup water, divided

1. Place watercress, tomatoes, celery, lemon, horseradish, cayenne, and 1/2 cup water in a blender and blend until thoroughly combined.
2. Add remaining 1/2 cup water while blending until desired texture is achieved.

Per Serving

Calorie 47| Fats 1g | Carbs 10g | Protein 2g

Homemade Golden Quiche

Prep time: 20 minutes | Cook time: 30 minutes | Serves 8

6 large eggs
6 slices nitrate-free bacon
1/2 cup chopped broccoli

1/2 cup sliced mushrooms
1/2 cup diced onions
1/2 cup diced red bell peppers

1. Preheat oven to 325°F.
2. Line up muffin tin with eight foil cups.
3. Whisk six eggs and set aside.
4. Cook bacon until crisp, drain on paper towels, and chop into 1/2" pieces.
5. Spray a medium sauté pan with cooking spray.
6. Sauté the remaining ingredients for 5 minutes
7. Pour eggs into foil cups, filling each two-thirds of the way.
8. Add bacon and vegetables to each cup.
9. Bake for 25 minutes or until golden brown.

Per Serving

Calorie 95| Fats 6g | Carbs 2g | Protein 7g

Peppery Lettuce Chicken Roll

Prep time: 20 minutes | Cook time: 0 minutes | Serves 3

2 pounds boneless, skinless chicken breast (baked, poached, or broiled)
2 medium stalks celery, chopped
1/4 cup chopped basil
2 tablespoons olive oil
2 tablespoons lemon juice
1 teaspoon minced garlic
1/8 teaspoon ground black pepper
8 large romaine lettuce leaves

1. Shred or finely chop chicken and place in a medium bowl.
2. Mix chicken with celery, basil, olive oil, lemon juice, garlic, and black pepper.
3. Separate lettuce leaves and place on eight plates.
4. Spoon chicken mixtures onto lettuce leaves and roll up.

Per Serving

Calorie 234| Fats 9g | Carbs 2g | Protein 36g

Mushroom- Bacon Egg fills

Prep time: 20 minutes | Cook time: 10 minutes | Serves 2

6 slices nitrate-free bacon, diced
1 medium yellow summer squash, chopped
1 cup sliced mushrooms
1 medium zucchini, chopped
1/4 cup fresh basil leaves, diced
2 tablespoons olive oil
8 large eggs, beaten

1. In a large sauté pan, cook bacon until crispy.
2. Add the vegetables and basil to the pan and sauté until tender, approximately 5–8 minutes.
3. Heat olive oil in a second large sauté pan over medium heat.
4. Cook eggs for 3 minutes on each side.
5. Place the vegetable and bacon mixture on one half of the eggs and fold over the other half to enclose the filling. Serve.

Per Serving

Calorie 584| Fats 44g | Carbs 9g | Protein 37g

Black pepper spiced Avocado with Baked Eggs

Prep time: 20 minutes | Cook time: 15 minutes | Serves 2

Medium or large avocados, halved and pitted
4 large eggs
¼ Teaspoon freshly ground black pepper

1. Preheat the oven to 220°C.
2. Scoop out some of the pulp from the avocado halves, leaving enough space to fit an egg, reserving the pulp for Easy Guacamole
3. Line an 8-by-8-inch baking pan with foil. Place the avocado halves in the pan to fit snugly in a single layer, folding the foil around the outer avocados to prevent tipping.
4. Crack 1 egg into each avocado half; season with pepper.
5. Bake, uncovered, until the whites are set and the egg yolks are cooked to your desired doneness, 12 to 15 minutes.
6. Remove from the oven and let rest for 5 minutes before serving.

Per Serving

Calorie 433| Fats 34 g| Carbs 16g| Protein 16.g

Goat Cheesed Peppery Scrambled Eggs

Prep time: 15 minutes | Cook time: 5 minutes | Serves 2

2 large eggs
1/8 teaspoon black pepper
1 teaspoon dried dill
weed
1 tablespoon crumbled goat cheese

1. Beat the eggs in a bowl; pour them into a nonstick skillet over medium heat.
2. Add black pepper and dill weed to eggs.
3. Cook until eggs are scrambled.
4. Top with crumbled goat cheese before serving.

Per Serving

Calorie 157| Fats 12.33g | Carbs 3.37g | Protein 8.14g

Very veggie Cauliflower Potato Hash

Prep time: 20 minutes | Cook time: 15 minutes | Serves 4

2 tablespoons coconut oil
2 large sweet potatoes, peeled and diced
3 Tablespoons water
1 small yellow onion, chopped
1 cup chopped cauliflower florets.
1 cup diced mushrooms
Salt and pepper to taste

1. Heat the coconut oil in a large skillet hot over medium-high heat.
2. Add the sweet potatoes, tossing to coat with oil, then add the water. Cover and simmer until the sweet potatoes are tender, about 8 to 10 minutes.
3. Stir in the onion, cauliflower and mushrooms. Cook for another 4 to 6 minutes until the onion is translucent.
4. Season with salt and pepper to taste and serve.

Per Serving

Calorie 210| Fats 7g| Carbs 35g| Protein 3g

Peppery Sweet Potato and Scrambled Eggs

Prep time: 20 minutes | Cook time: 15 minutes | Serves 6

2 tablespoons coconut oil
3 medium sweet potatoes, peeled and grated
1 tablespoon grass-fed butter
6 large eggs
1/4 teaspoon salt
1/8 teaspoon ground black pepper

1. Heat coconut oil in a large skillet over medium-high heat.
2. Cook sweet potatoes in hot oil for 7 minutes, stirring often. Drain on paper towels.
3. Meanwhile, in a medium skillet, heat butter over medium heat.
4. Pour in eggs and cook until no visible liquid egg remains, stirring occasionally.
5. Season with salt and black pepper.
6. To serve, top the Sweet Potato Hash Browns with Scrambled egg.

Per Serving

Calorie 186| Fats 12g | Carbs 12g | Protein 8g

Homemade Apple Cinnamon Oat Meal

Prep time: 15 minutes | Cook time: 10 minutes | Serves 2

1/3 cup quick-cooking oatmeal
1 large egg
1/2 cup almond milk
1/4 teaspoon cinnamon
1/2 medium apple

1. Core and finely chop apple half.
2. Combine oats, egg and almond milk in a large mug. Stir well with a fork.
3. Add cinnamon and apple. Stir again until fully mixed.
4. Cook in microwave on high for 2 minutes. Fluff with a fork. Cook an additional 30 to 60 seconds if needed.
5. Stir in a little more milk or water if thinner cereal is desired.

Per Serving

Calorie 261| Fats 10.86g | Carbs 31.38g | Protein 10.81g

Butter Egg omelet with Pepper

Prep time: 5 minutes | Cook time: 10 minutes | Serves 2

1 tablespoon unable salted butter, cooled
4 large eggs
Table salt and pepper

1. Heat 10-inch nonstick skillet over low heat for 5 minutes.
2. Meanwhile, crack open 2 eggs into mug or small pot: crack remaining 2 eggs into second mug or small pot.
3. Insert butter to skillet, let melt, and swirl to coat dish.
4. Pour 2 eggs into skillet on one side and remaining 2 eggs on opposite side.
5. Season eggs with table salt and pepper to taste, wrap up, and prepare about 2 minutes for runny yolks, 3 minutes for soft but set yolks, or 3 minutes for firmly set yolks.
6. Slide eggs onto plate; serve.

Per Serving

Calorie 305| Fats 25.82g | Carbs 6.91g | Protein 11.54g

Chicken Cucumber Tomato Salad

Prep time: 15 minutes | Cook time: 0 minutes | Serves 2

4 ounces rotisserie chicken, roughly sliced off
4 Tablespoon extra-virgin olive oil
½ scallion, sliced off
1-ounce favourite greens
1-ounce red bell pepper, sliced off
1-ounce cherry tomatoes, halved
1-ounce cucumber, sliced off
Table salt and black pepper to the taste

1. In a pot, combine greens with bell pepper, tomatoes, scallion, cucumber, table salt, pepper and olive oil and fling to coat well.
2. Shift this to a jar, top with chicken pieces and serve for breakfast.

Per Serving

Calorie 520| Fats 41.45g | Carbs 13.7g | Protein 23.98g

Thyme flavoured baked Eggs with Asparagus and Tomatoes

Prep time: 30 minutes | Cook time: 20 minutes | Serves 2

4 eggs
2 tablespoons olive oil
907 g asparagus
1-pint cherry tomatoes
2 Teaspoons chopped fresh thyme
Salt and pepper to taste

1. Preheat the oven to 400°F. Grease a baking sheet with non-stick cooking spray.
2. Arrange the asparagus and cherry tomatoes in an even layer on the baking sheet.
3. Drizzle the olive oil over the vegetables; season with the thyme and salt and pepper to taste.
4. Roast in the oven until the asparagus is nearly tender and the tomatoes are wrinkled, 10 to 12 minutes.
5. Crack the eggs on top of the asparagus; season each with salt and pepper.
6. Return to the oven and bake until the egg whites are set but the yolks are still jiggly, 7 to 8 minutes more.
7. To serve, divide the asparagus, tomatoes and eggs among four plates.

Per Serving

Calorie 158 | Fats 13g| Carbs 11g| Protein 11g

Baked Spicy pepper Muffins

Prep time: 30 minutes | Cook time: 20 minutes | Serves 2

Extra-virgin olive oil, coconut oil, or clarified butter, for greasing (optional)
12 large eggs
2 Teaspoons sea salt or Himalayan salt
2 Teaspoons freshly ground black pepper
1 medium red bell pepper, seeded and diced
1 medium orange, yellow, or green bell pepper, seeded and diced
1 cup packed baby spinach, finely chopped
½ cup thinly sliced scallions
1 small jalapeño pepper, seeded and minced (optional)

1. Preheat the oven to 180°C. Grease a 12-hole muffin pan or use paper muffin liners.
2. In a large bowl, place the eggs, salt, and pepper and beat until fluffy. Add the peppers, spinach, scallions, and jalapeño, stirring to combine.
3. Ladle the egg mixture evenly into the prepared muffin pan.
4. Bake until a toothpick or paring knife comes out clean when inserted, about 20 minutes. Let the muffins cool in the pan about 10 minutes before serving.

Per Serving

Calorie 82| Fats 6 g| Carbs 2g| Protein 2 g

Cheesy Toasted Golden Bagel with Tomato

Prep time: 15 minutes | Cook time: 5 minutes | Serves 2

1 bagel, 2-ounce size
2 tablespoons cream cheese
2 tomato slices, 1/4" thick
2 red onion slices
1 teaspoon low-sodium lemon pepper seasoning

1. Slice bagel and toast until golden brown.
2. Spread cream cheese over each bagel half.
3. Place onion slice and tomato slice on top and sprinkle with lemon pepper.

Per Serving

Calorie 177| Fats 9.1g | Carbs 19.15g | Protein 5.54g

Walnut Pumpkin Pancake

Prep time: 10 minutes |Cook time: 3 minutes |Serves 5

1 1/3 cups pumpkin puree	1 Teaspoon ground cinnamon
6 large eggs, whisked	1/4 Teaspoon ground nutmeg
1/2 cup plus 1 Tablespoon coconut flour	Pinch salt
2 tablespoons pure maple syrup	1/2 cup chopped walnuts (optional)

1. Heat a large non-stick skillet over medium heat. In a food processor, combine the pumpkin, eggs, maple syrup and vanilla extract.
2. Blend smooth then pulse in the coconut flour, cinnamon, nutmeg and salt. Spoon the batter into the hot skillet, using about 3 Tablespoons per pancake.
3. Sprinkle a few chopped walnuts into the wet batter and cook for 1 to 2 minutes until the underside is browned. Flip the pancakes and cook for another minute or two until browned on the underside.
4. Transfer the pancakes to a plate to keep warm and repeat with the remaining batter.

Per Serving

Calorie 250| Fats 15g| Carbs 19g| Protein 13 g

Lemony Avocado Salman Wraps

Prep time: 10 minutes | Cook time: 0 minutes | Serves 2

4 large romaine lettuce leaves	4 ounces smoked salmon, cut into four equal pieces
1 large avocado, pitted, peeled, and sliced	Juice of 1 medium lemon

1. Arrange lettuce leaves on two plates.
2. Stack avocado slices and salmon on top of lettuce leaves. Sprinkle with lemon juice.
3. Fold lettuce leaves in half and serve.

Per Serving

Calorie 195| Fats 13g | Carbs 9g | Protein 13g

Maple Walnut Almond Granola

Prep time: 30 minutes | Cook time: 25 minutes | Serves 2

1½ cups chopped raw walnuts or pecans	unsalted grass-fed butter, melted
1 cup raw almonds, sliced	1 Tablespoon maple syrup
½ cup seeds, toasted or roasted unsalted sunflower, sesame, or shelled pumpkin	1 Teaspoon alcohol-free vanilla extract
¼ cup unsweetened coconut flakes	1 Teaspoon ground cinnamon, or to taste
½ cup coconut oil or	¼ Teaspoon sea salt or Himalayan salt

1. Preheat the oven to 150°C.
2. Line a rimmed baking sheet with parchment paper or foil.
3. Add the walnuts, almonds, seeds, and coconut flakes to a large bowl.
4. In a separate bowl, mix the oil with the maple syrup, vanilla, cinnamon, and salt. Pour over the nut mixture, tossing to coat.
5. Spread the mixture evenly on the prepared baking sheet and bake until golden brown, about 25 minutes, stirring once halfway through. Cool completely.

Per Serving

Calorie 248 | Fats 25g| Carbs 6g| Protein 4g

Frozen cherries and coconut milk smoothie

Prep time: 15 minutes | Cook time: 0 minutes | Serves 2

1 mug water	coconut milk
1 mug cherries, frozen	1 mug favorite greens
¼ mug cocoa grinding grains	¼ mug cocoa nibs
10 ounces canned	1 small avocado, pitted and peeled
	¼ Teaspoon. turmeric

1. In your blender, combine coconut milk with avocado, cocoa grinding grains, cherries and turmeric and blend well.
2. Add water, greens and cocoa nibs, blend for 2 minutes more, pour into glasses and serve.

Per Serving

Calorie 378| Fats 30.06g | Carbs 28.2g | Protein 6.14g

Almond and carrot Superhero Muffins

Prep time: 20 minutes | Cook time: 20 minutes | Serves 12

2 cups almond flour
1 Teaspoon ground cinnamon
1 Teaspoon baking soda
1/2 Teaspoon ground ginger
1/4 Teaspoon salt

3 large eggs, whisked well
1/2 cup unsweetened applesauce
1/2 cup pure maple syrup
1 cup fresh grated carrots

1. Preheat the oven to 350°F and line a muffin pan with paper liners.
2. Combine the dry ingredients in a large mixing bowl and stir well.
3. In a separate bowl, beat together the eggs, applesauce and maple syrup. Stir the carrot into the wet ingredients then stir the mixture into the dry ingredients.
4. Spoon the batter into the muffin pan, filling the cups 2/3 full. Bake for 18 to 20 minutes until a knife inserted in the centre comes out clean.

Per Serving
Calorie 90| Fats 4g| Carbs 12g| Protein 3g

Sugar free Blueberry Banana Pancakes

Prep time: 20 minutes |Cook time: 10 minutes |Serves 12 pancakes

1 overripe banana
2 large eggs
1 Tablespoon alcohol-free vanilla extract
1 Teaspoon ground cinnamon
Pinch sea salt or

Himalayan salt
¼ cup coconut oil or clarified butter, divided
2 cups fresh or frozen blueberries

1. In a medium bowl, mash the banana until softened.
2. Add the eggs and continue to mash until smooth and most of the chunks are blended. Stir in the vanilla, cinnamon, and salt.
3. Heat 1 Tablespoon of the coconut oil in a large skillet or flat cast iron pan over medium heat.

4. Pour in 2 to 3 Tablespoons of the batter to form 3-inch rounds. Cook the pancakes four at a time until set and golden brown, 2 to 4 minutes total, flipping once and transfer to a plate to cool and repeat until the remaining batter is used up, adding 1 Tablespoon coconut oil in between each batch.
5. In a separate, small saucepan, add the blueberries and remaining 1 Tablespoon coconut oil. Cook over medium heat, constantly mashing berries with a wooden spoon, until juices reduce to a syrup-like consistency, 3 to 5 minutes and Set aside to cool.
6. Serve pancakes with the blueberry syrup on the side.

Per Serving
Calorie 224 | Fats 17g| Carbs 18g| Protein 16g

Oven Baked Asparagus with Eggs and Tomatoes

Prep time: 30 minutes | Cook time: 20 minutes | Serves 2

4 eggs
2 tablespoons olive oil
2 Teaspoons chopped fresh thyme
907 g asparagus

1-pint cherry tomatoes
Salt and pepper to taste

1. Preheat the oven to 400°F and grease a baking sheet with non-stick cooking spray.
2. Arrange the asparagus and cherry tomatoes in an even layer on the baking sheet.
3. Drizzle the olive oil over the vegetables; season with the thyme and salt and pepper to taste.
4. Roast in the oven until the asparagus is nearly tender and the tomatoes are wrinkled, 10 to 12 minutes.
5. Crack the eggs on top of the asparagus; season each with salt and pepper.
6. Return to the oven and bake until the egg whites are set but the yolks are still jiggly, 7 to 8 minutes more.
7. Divide the asparagus, tomatoes and eggs among four plates, to serve.

Per Serving
Calorie 158 | Fats11 g| Carbs13 g| Protein 11g

Healthy Coconut Granola

Prep time: 30 minutes | Cook time: 20 minutes | Serves 16

2 cups unsweetened coconut flakes
2 cups slivered almonds
1 cup chopped macadamia nuts
1 cup broken walnuts
1/2 cup sesame seeds
1/2 cup pumpkin seeds
1 cup golden raisins
1 cup dried unsweetened cranberries
1 cup chopped Medjool dates
1 teaspoon cinnamon
1 teaspoon ground ginger
1/2 teaspoon nutmeg
8 cups unsweetened vanilla almond milk

1. In a large bowl, combine all ingredients except milk and mix well. Store in an airtight container at room temperature for up to a few weeks.
2. To serve, pour 1 cup muesli into a small serving bowl and add 1 cup almond milk. Let stand for 5 minutes before eating.
3. You can also make this muesli the night before. Place muesli in a large bowl and cover with milk or water.
4. Cover and let stand overnight in the refrigerator. When you're ready to eat breakfast, stir the muesli and dig in.

Per Serving
Calorie 370| Fats 26g | Carbs 30g | Protein 9g

Breakfast Cranberry and Almond porridge

Prep time: 30 minutes | Cook time: 120 minutes | Serves 16

1/2 cup dried cranberries
1/4 cup slivered almonds
1/4 cup raw pumpkin seeds
1/4 cup raw sunflower seeds
1/4 cup unsweetened shredded coconut
1/8 cup maple syrup
2 tablespoons grass-fed butter, melted

1. Line a baking sheet with parchment paper and set aside.
2. Place dried cranberries, almonds, pumpkin seeds, sunflower seeds, and coconut in a 4-quart slow cooker. Add maple syrup and butter and toss to coat.

3. Cover (but vent with a chopstick) and cook on high for 21/2–31/2 hours, stirring periodically to prevent burning.
4. Cool porridge by spreading it out in a single layer on lined baking sheet. Store in the refrigerator in a tightly sealed container for up to several days. Serve warm

Per Serving
Calorie 206| Fats 14g | Carbs 19g | Protein 4g

Healthy Roasted Nuts and seeds

Prep time: 30 minutes | Cook time: 20 minutes | Serves 2

11/2 cups pumpkin seeds
1 cup sunflower seeds
11/2 cups sliced almonds
11/2 cups chopped pecans
11/2 cups unsweetened shredded coconut
1/3 cup maple syrup
1/3 cup coconut oil
1 teaspoon cinnamon
2 teaspoons vanilla
1 cup dried cranberries
1 cup chopped dried apricots
1 cup golden raisins

1. Preheat oven to 375°F. Line a rimmed baking sheet with parchment paper and set aside.
2. In a large bowl, combine pumpkin seeds, sunflower seeds, almonds, pecans, and coconut. Spread mixture onto lined baking sheet.
3. In a small saucepan, combine maple syrup and coconut oil and heat gently until coconut oil is melted.
4. Remove from heat and stir in cinnamon and vanilla.
5. Drizzle over the mixture on baking sheet and toss to coat. Spread evenly.
6. Bake for 20–30 minutes, stirring every 10 minutes, until light golden brown and fragrant.
7. Remove from oven and stir in cranberries, apricots, and raisins.
8. Let stand until cool, stirring occasionally.
9. Store in an airtight container at room temperature for few weeks.

Per Serving
Calorie 351| Fats 26g | Carbs 27g | Protein 8g

Best Pumpkin cake ever

Prep time: 30 minute | Cook time: 40 minute | Serves 2

11/2 cups pumpkin seeds
1/2 cup solid-pack canned pumpkin
1/2 cup puréed canned pears
2 large eggs
3/4 cup maple syrup
1/4 cup canned full-fat coconut milk
1 teaspoon vanilla
1 cup almond flour
3/4 cup coconut flour
2 tablespoons arrowroot powder
1/2 teaspoon salt
1/8 teaspoon baking soda
1/4 teaspoon cream of tartar
1/2 teaspoon cinnamon
1/4 teaspoon nutmeg
1/4 teaspoon cardamom

1. Preheat oven to 350°F. Line a 9" × 5" loaf pan with parchment paper and set aside.
2. In a large bowl, combine pumpkin, pears, eggs, maple syrup, coconut milk, and vanilla and beat well.
3. In a medium bowl, stir together almond flour, coconut flour, arrowroot powder, salt, baking soda, cream of tartar, cinnamon, nutmeg, and cardamom.
4. Add the dry ingredients to the pumpkin mixture and mix well. Pour into prepared loaf pan.
5. Bake for 40–50 minutes or until a toothpick inserted in the centre comes out clean. Cool in pan for 15 minutes, then remove loaf and move to a wire rack to cool completely.

Per Serving
Calorie 127| Fats 6g | Carbs 17g | Protein 3g

Poached Apple and Pears with Cinnamon

Prep time: 20 minutes | Cook time: 120 minutes | Serves 5

2 medium Granny Smith apples, peeled, cored, and halved (save cores)
2 medium Bartlett pears, peeled, cored, and halved (save cores)
1 large orange, peeled, seeded, and halved
2/3 cup maple syrup
1 vanilla bean, split and seeded (save seeds)
1 cinnamon stick

1. Place apple and pear cores in a 41/2-quart slow cooker.
2. Squeeze juice from orange halves into the slow cooker and add orange halves, maple syrup, vanilla bean and seeds, and cinnamon stick.
3. Add apples and pears and pour in enough water to cover the fruit. Stir, cover, and cook on high for 2–3 hours, until fruit is tender.
4. Remove apple and pear halves and set aside.
5. Strain cooking liquids into a large saucepan and simmer gently over low heat until liquid reduces by half and thickens. Discard solids.
6. Dice apples and pears and add to saucepan to warm.
7. To serve, spoon fruit with sauce into small serving bowls.

Per Serving
Calorie 127| Fats 6g | Carbs 17g | Protein 3g

Garlic roasted Brussels sprouts with pepper

Prep time: 30 minutes | Cook time: 15 minutes | Serves 5

4-6 slices nitrate free bacon
Salt and pepper
1 lb. Brussels sprouts halved (or quartered for larger ones)
4 cloves garlic minced
2 tablespoons balsamic vinegar

1. Preheat your oven to 425 degrees.
2. Spread Brussels sprouts in a single layer on a large baking sheet.
3. Cut bacon into pieces, then sprinkle all over Brussels sprouts.
4. Roast in the preheated oven for 15 mins, then stir and return to a single layer and continue to roast another 5-10 mins until bacon is crisp.
5. Drizzle all over with vinegar and sprinkle with the garlic.
6. Continue to roast another 5-7 mins or until browned and crispy.
7. Serve as a side dish anytime! Enjoy!

Per Serving
Calorie 82| Fats 6g| Carbs 2g| Protein 2g

Peaches Crisp with Almond and coconut flakes

Prep time: 15 minutes | Cook time: 30 minutes | Serves 2

½ Teaspoon. Ground cinnamon
1 mug unsweetened coconut flakes
1 mug coarsely sliced off raw almonds
¼ mug unable salted raw sunflower seeds
1 tablespoon fresh lemon juice
6 ripe peaches
½ mug unsweetened, unsulfured dried

peaches, finely sliced off
¾ mug fresh orange juice
¼ mug unrefined coconut oil
1 vanilla bean, split and seeds scraped
1 mug raspberries, blueberries, blackberries, and/ or coarsely sliced off strawberries

1. In a huge sauce dish bring 8 mugs water to bubbling. Utilizing a sharp blade, cut a shallow X on the lower part of each peach.
2. Drench peaches, two all at once, in bubbling water for 30 to 60 seconds or until skins start to part.
3. Utilizing an opened spoon, move peaches to an enormous pot of ice water. At the point when sufficiently cool to deal with, utilize a blade or your fingers to strip off skins; eliminate skins.
4. Cut peaches into wedges, eliminating the pits; put in a safe spot. Preheat broiler to 250°F.
5. Line a huge preparing sheet with material paper.
6. In a food processor or blender consolidate 1 cup of the peach wedges, the dried peaches, ¼ cup of the squeezed orange, the coconut oil, and cinnamon.
7. Wrap up and cycle or mix until smooth; put in a safe spot. In an enormous pot join the coconut pieces, almonds, and sunflower seeds.
8. Addition pureed peach join. Throw to cover. Move nut consolidate to the readied heating sheet, Scattering equally.
9. Prepare for 25 to 30 minutes or until dry and fresh, shake ring at times. (Be mindful so as not to consume; join will fresh up additional as it cools.)
10. Meanwhile, Put the leftover peach wedges into a moderate substantial sauce dish.
11. Shake in the excess ½ mug squeezed orange, the lemon squeeze, and split vanilla bean (with seeds).
12. Bring to bubbling over moderate warmth, shake ring once in a while. Lessen warmth to low; stew, open up increased, for 10 to 15 minutes or until thickened, shake ring every so often.
13. Eliminate vanilla bean unit. Shake in berries. Get ready for 3 to 4 minutes or just until berries are warmed through.

Per Serving
Calorie 32| Fats 7.9g | Carbs 6.41g | Protein 8.5

Rice Milk Blueberry Muffins

Prep time: 15 minutes | Cook time: 30 minutes | Serves 2

2 cups unsweetened rice milk
1 tablespoon apple cider vinegar
3½ cups all-purpose flour
1 cup granulated sugar
1 tablespoon Ener-G baking soda substitute

1 teaspoon ground cinnamon
½ teaspoon ground nutmeg
Pinch ground ginger
½ cup canola oil
2 tablespoons pure vanilla extract
2½ cups fresh blueberries

1. Preheat the oven to 375°F.
2. Line the cups of a muffin pan with paper liners; set aside.
3. In a small bowl, stir together the rice milk and vinegar; set aside for 10 minutes.
4. In a large bowl, stir together the flour, sugar, baking soda substitute,
5. Cinnamon, nutmeg, and ginger until well mixed. Add the oil and vanilla to the milk mixture and stir to blend.
6. Add the milk mixture to the dry ingredients and stir until just combined.
7. Fold in the blueberries. Spoon the muffin batter evenly into the cups.
8. Bake the muffins for 25 to 30 minutes or until golden and a toothpick
9. Inserted in the centre of a muffin comes out clean.
10. Allow the muffins to cool for 15 minutes before serving.

Per Serving
Calorie 3896| Fats 131.8g | Carbs 604g | Protein 64.91g

Peppery Egg with Italian Bread

Prep time: 15 minutes | Cook time: 5 minutes | Serves 2

2 (½-inch-thick) slices Italian bread
¼ cup unsalted butter
2 eggs
2 tablespoons

chopped fresh chives
Pinch cayenne pepper
Freshly ground black pepper

1. Using a cookie cutter or a small glass cut a 2-inch round from the center of each piece of bread.
2. In a large nonstick skillet over medium-high heat, melt the butter.
3. Place the bread in the skillet, toast it for 1 minute, and then flip the bread over.
4. Crack the eggs into the holes the Centre of the bread and cook for about 2 minutes or until the eggs are set and the bread is golden brown.
5. Top with chopped chives, cayenne pepper, and black pepper.
6. Cook the bread for another 2 minutes.
7. Transfer an egg-in-the-hole to each plate to serve.

Per Serving
Calorie 649| Fats 51.58g | Carbs 22.9g | Protein 23.5g

Scallion parsley Egg Omelet

Prep time: 15 minutes | Cook time: 10 minutes | Serves 2

4 egg whites
1 egg
2 tablespoons chopped fresh parsley
2 tablespoons water
Olive oil spray, for greasing the skillet

½ cup chopped and boiled red bell pepper
¼ cup chopped scallion, both green and white parts
Freshly ground black pepper

1. In a small bowl, whisk together the egg whites, egg, parsley, and water until well blended; set aside.
2. Generously spray a large nonstick skillet with olive oil spray and place it over medium-high heat.
3. Sauté the peppers and scallion for about 3 minutes or until softened.
4. Pour the egg mixture into the skillet over the vegetables and cook, swirling

5. the skillet, for about 2 minutes or until the edges of the egg start to set.
6. Lift up the set edges and tilt the pan so that the uncooked egg can flow underneath the cooked egg.
7. Continue lifting and cooking the egg for about 4 minutes or until the omelet is set.
8. Loosen the omelet with a spatula and fold it in half. Cut the folded omelet into 3 portions and transfer the omelets to serving plates.
9. Season with black pepper and serve.

Per Serving
Calorie 220| Fats 10.09g | Carbs 6.53g | Protein 24.68g

Spicy Rice milk Egg Muffins

Prep time: 15 minutes | Cook time: 10 minutes | Serves 2

Cooking spray, for greasing the muffin pans
4 eggs
2 tablespoons unsweetened rice milk
½ sweet onion, finely chopped

½ red bell pepper, finely chopped
1 tablespoon chopped fresh parsley
Pinch red pepper flakes
Pinch freshly ground black pepper

1. Preheat the oven to 350°F.
2. Spray 4 muffin pans with cooking spray; set aside.
3. In a large bowl, whisk together the eggs, milk, onion, red pepper, parsley,
4. red pepper flakes, and black pepper until well combined.
5. Pour the egg mixture into the prepared muffin pans.
6. Bake 18 to 20 minutes or until the muffins are puffed and golden.
7. Serve warm or cold.

Per Serving
Calorie 618| Fats 39.83g | Carbs 24.62g | Protein 39.6g

Peppery Eggs with Lemon Hollandaise Sauce

Prep time: 18 minutes | Cook time: 15 minutes | Serves 2

Hollandia Sauce:

3 large egg yolks (save whites for other use)	1 Tablespoon lemon juice (from about ½ lemons)
½ cup extra-virgin olive oil, ghee, or clarified butter	Pinch salt Pinch cayenne pepper

Eggs:

2 Teaspoons apple cider vinegar or white vinegar	ends removed, cut into 4 thick slices
4 large eggs	1 cup baby spinach
1 large ripe beefsteak or heirloom tomato	Freshly ground black pepper

1. For the hollandaise sauce, bring a pot of water, filled to about 4 inches up the sides, to a boil.
2. Set aside 2 tablespoons of the hot water.
3. In a medium metal bowl, whisk the egg yolks.
4. Add in the olive oil, hot water, lemon juice, salt, and cayenne and continue whisking.
5. Hover the bowl over the pot of boiling water. Whisk constantly until the sauce thickens, 1 to 2 minutes, keeping the bowl from touching the boiling water, to prevent the eggs from curdling.
6. Remove the bowl of hollandaise sauce from the pot of water, and set it aside on another part of the stovetop.
7. To poach the eggs, reduce the heat under the pot of boiling water to a simmer and add the vinegar.
8. Prepare a paper-towel lined plate.
9. One at a time, carefully crack the eggs into a small bowl, and then use the bowl to slowly slide 2 of the eggs into the water. Simmer for 2 minutes.
10. Using a slotted spoon, transfer the eggs to the paper towel-lined plate. Repeat the process with the remaining 2 eggs.
11. To serve, divide the tomato slices between two plates.
12. Top each tomato with a few spinach leaves, 1 poached egg, and 2 heaping Tablespoons of the warm hollandaise.
13. Season with black pepper and serve immediately.

Per Serving
Calorie 423| Fats 39g| Carbs 6g| Protein 16g

Buttery Veg Egg Mix with Pita Bread

Prep time: 15 minutes | Cook time: 5 minutes | Serves 2

3 eggs, beaten	½ teaspoon ground ginger
1 scallion, both green and white parts, finely chopped	2 tablespoons light sour cream
½ red bell pepper, finely chopped	2 (4-inch) plain pita bread pockets, halved
2 teaspoons unsalted butter	½ cup julienned English cucumber
1 teaspoon curry powder	1 cup roughly chopped watercress

1. In a small bowl, whisk together the eggs, scallion, and red pepper until well blended.
2. In a large nonstick skillet over medium heat, melt the butter.
3. Pour the egg mixture into the skillet and cook for about 3 minutes or until
4. the eggs are just set, swirling the skillet but not stirring.
5. Remove the eggs from the heat; set aside.
6. In a small bowl, stir together the curry powder, ginger, and sour cream until well blended.
7. Evenly divide the curry sauce among the 4 halves of the pita bread, spreading it out on one inside edge.
8. Divide the cucumber and watercress evenly between the halves.
9. Spoon the eggs into the halves, dividing the mixture evenly, to serve.

Per Serving
Calorie 1005| Fats 58.36g | Carbs 40.95g | Protein 75.27g

Instant Moist Eggs with scallion greens

Prep time: 10 minutes | Cook time: 10 minutes | Serves 2

12 large eggs
1 Teaspoon. Vegetable oil
8 ounces sweet Italian sausage, casings removed, sausage crumbled into 1 -inch pieces
1 red bell pepper, stemmed, seeded, and slice into 1 -inch pieces
3 scallions, white and green parts separated, both sliced thin on bias
6 Tablespoon half-and-half
3/ 4 Teaspoon. table salt
1 Teaspoon. pepper
1 tablespoon unable salted butter
11 ounces sharp cheddar cheese, shredded (1 mug)

1. Beat eggs, half-and-half, table salt, and pepper with fork in moderate pot until thoroughly combined.
2. Heat oil in 12-inch non-stick skillet over moderate heat until shimmering. Insert sausage and prepare, breaking into 1 -inch pieces until beginning to brown, about 2 minutes.
3. Insert bell pepper and scallion whites; continue to prepare, shake ring occasionally, until sausage is prepared through and pepper is beginning to brown, about 3 minutes.
4. Scatters combine in single layer on moderate plate; set aside.
5. Wipe out skillet with paper towels.
6. Insert butter to now-empty skillet and melt over moderate heat, swirling to coat dish.
7. Pour in egg combine.
8. With heatproof rubber spatula, shake eggs constantly, slowly pushing them from side to side, scraping along bottom and sides of skillet, and lifting and folding eggs as they form curds (do not over scramble or curds formed will be too small).
9. Prepare until large curds form but eggs are still very moist, 2 to 3 minutes.
10. Off heat, gently fold in sausage combine and cheddar until evenly distributed; if eggs are still underdone, return skillet to moderate heat for no longer than 30 seconds.
11. Distribute eggs among individual plates, Garnish with scallion greens, and serve instantly.

Per Serving
Calorie 1213| Fats 87.98g | Carbs 31.39g | Protein 73.25g

Salmon Egg Sandwich with Avocado

Prep time: 15 minutes | Cook time: 10 minutes | Serves 2

2 Tablespoon thinly sliced scallions
1 Teaspoon black pepper
10 ounces prepared salmon
2 egg whites
½ mug almond flour
⅓ mug shredded sweet potato
4 Tablespoon olive oil
2 Tablespoon snipped fresh cilantro
2 Tablespoon Chipotle Paleo Mayo
1 tablespoon fresh lime juice
1 ripe avocado, peeled, seeded, and sliced

1. For salmon patties, at a large pot using a Fork to flake grilled salmon into little pieces. Combine lightly to blend.
2. Distribute combined into eight parts.
3. Shape each portion into a patty. (Cakes could be cooled 1 day before serving.)
4. Heat 2 tablespoon of olive oil in a large nonstick skillet on moderate-immense heat. Insert half of those cakes into the skillet.
5. Prepare about 8 minutes or till golden brown, turning the cakes halfway through preparing.
6. Shift the cakes into a different parchment-lined baking sheet and keep warm from the oven.
7. Fry the rest of the cakes at the remaining 2 tablespoons oil as directed.
8. To serve, Organize Zucchini Ribbons at a nest on all four serving dishes. Top each with two salmon sandwiches, a poached egg, a number of those Tomatillo-Mango Salsa, and avocado slices

Per Serving
Calorie 1382| Fats 114.19g | Carbs 23.51g | Protein 70.41g

Spiced Trout with Smoky seasoning

Prep time: 15 minute | Cook time: 10 minute | Serves 2

3 Tablespoon refined coconut oil
1½ pounds white or yellow sweet potatoes, peeled
Refined coconut oil for frying
Sliced off fresh parsley
4 6ounce fresh or

frozen skinless trout fillets, ¼ to ½ inch thick
1½ teaspoons Smoky Seasoning
¼ to ½ Teaspoon. black pepper (optional)
Sliced scallions

1. Preheat oven to 400°F. Thaw fish, if frozen. Rinse fish; pat dry with paper towels.
2. Garnish fillets with Smoky Seasoning and, if desired, pepper. In an extra-large oven going skillet heat 2 Tablespoon of the oil over moderate-immense heat.
3. Put fillets in skillet and bake, unwrap upped, for 6 to 8 minutes or until fish begins to flake when tested with a fork.
4. Remove from oven. Meanwhile, using a julienne peeler or mandolin fitted with the julienne slicer, slice sweet potatoes lengthwise into long thin strips.
5. Wrap potato strips in a double thickness of paper towels and absorb any excess water.
6. In a large stockpot with at least 8-inch-tall sides, heat 2 to 3 inches of refined coconut oil to 365°F.
7. Carefully insert potatoes, about one-fourth at a time, to the warm oil. (Oil will rise in the pot.)
8. Fry about 1 to 3 minutes per batch or until just starting to brown, shake ring once or twice.
9. Quickly remove potatoes using a long-slotted spoon and drain on paper towels. (Potatoes can over prepare quickly, so check early and often.) Be sure to heat oil back up to 365°F before inserting each batch of potatoes.
10. Garnish trout with parsley and scallions
11. Serve with sweet potato shoestrings.

Per Serving
Calorie 47| Fats 1g | Carbs 10g | Protein 2g

Spicy Garlicky Tomato Onion Omelet

Prep time: 30 minutes| Cook time: 10 minutes | serves: 6

1 bell pepper, diced
1 zucchini, diced
2 cloves garlic, minced
1 Tablespoon olive oil or 1/4 cup water (for water sauté)
2 medium potatoes, diced (with or without the skin)
1 small onion, diced
Handful grape tomatoes, halved or quartered
Pinch of red pepper flakes, optional

Mineral salt and fresh cracked pepper, to taste
1 Teaspoon mustard or 1/2 Teaspoon mustard powder
1 1/2 Teaspoons dried tarragon, thyme or basil
1/2 Teaspoon garlic powder
1/2 Teaspoon salt
1/4 Teaspoon turmeric
1/8 Teaspoon white or black pepper, optional

1. Preheat the oven to 375 degrees F.
2. In a pan, heats oil over medium heat, sauté potatoes for 5 minutes, add onion and cook for an additional 5 minutes.
3. Add bell pepper, zucchini and garlic, cook until softened. Add tomatoes and optional red pepper flakes, cook another minute or two. Season with salt and pepper to taste.
4. Combine the remaining ingredients in a food processor and process until smooth. Taste for seasoning.
5. Add the tofu mixture to the pan, the vegetables cooked in and mix well.
6. Spoon mixture into a lightly greased round pie/quiche dish or spring form pan.
7. Level the top flat with the back of a spatula or spoon and make sure all edges are filled.
8. Place on the middle rack and bake for 35 – 45 minutes, frittata should be firm to the touch. If the top starts to brown too much, cover with foil or a small silpat.
9. Remove and let stand to cool for at least 10 minutes. If using a pie/quiche dish, loosen the edges of the frittata, place a plate over top and carefully flip so the frittata falls onto the plate and serve (this step is optional).
10. This frittata is great with sliced avocado and a little sriracha for heat.

Per Serving
Calorie 226| Fats 9g| Carbs 22g| Protein 16g

CHAPTER 4: LUNCH RECIPES

Easy Veggie Turkey Mix

Prep time: 15 minute | Cook time: 20 minute | Serves 7

½ lbs. ground turkey
1/3 cup shredded carrots
1/3 cup shredded beets
1/3 cup zucchini
½ teaspoon garlic, minced
1 teaspoon onion,

minced
1 teaspoon ginger, minced
½ teaspoon brown sugar
½ teaspoon black pepper
½ teaspoon paprika

1. Mix together ground turkey, shredded carrots, shredded beets, shredded zucchini, minced garlic, minced onion, minced ginger, brown sugar, black pepper, paprika.
2. Using hands form into 3 oz. patties, grill over medium-high heat 4-5 minutes per side.

Per Serving

Calorie 464| Fats 17.87g| Carbs 30.74g| Protein 47.29g

Carrot and Onion Scrambled Egg

Prep time: 10 minute | Cook time: 5 minute | Serves 2

½ lb. carrot
1 tablespoon olive oil
½ red onions
¼ Teaspoon salt

2 oz. cheddar cheese
1 garlic clove
¼ Teaspoon dill
4Eggs

1. In a bowl whisk eggs with salt and cheese
2. In a frying pan heat olive oil and pour egg mixture
3. Add remaining ingredients and mix well
4. Serve when ready

Per Serving

Calorie 845| Fats 57.64g| Carbs 35.18g| Protein 46.07g

Lemony Quinoa Salad with Peppery Tuna

Prep time: 10 minute | Cook time: 10 minute | Serves 2

2/3 cup quinoa, prepared
½ tablespoon red pepper infused olive oil
½ can organic whole kernel corn drained
3 pickled beets, quartered

1 teaspoon toasted coriander seeds
6 pickled jalapenos
1 ripe avocado peeled and sliced
Juice of ½ lemon
2 filets tuna
Salt and pepper
¼ cup coconut oil

1. Preheat broiler and prepare 9x11 dishes.
2. In Dutch oven combine olive oil, corn, pickled beets, toasted coriander seeds, pickled jalapenos.
3. Toss with prepared quinoa and warm through.
4. Sprinkle Tunas with salt and pepper then brush both sides with coconut oil. Place under broiler 5 minutes per-ide.

Per Serving

Calorie 997| Fats 89.87g| Carbs 50.66g| Protein 10.48g

Simple Belgian endive Egg with Cheese and Onion

Prep time: 10 minute | Cook time: 5 minute | Serves 2

½ lb. Belgian endive
1 tablespoon olive oil
½ red onion
¼ Teaspoon salt

2 oz. cheddar cheese
1 garlic clove
¼ Teaspoon dill
4 Eggs

1. In a bowl whisk eggs with salt and cheese
2. In a frying pan heat olive oil and pour egg mixture
3. Add remaining ingredients and mix well
4. Serve when ready

Per Serving

Calorie 804| Fats 57.69g| Carbs 24.14g| Protein 47.18g

Spicy Coconut Sweet Potato with Kale

Prep time: 10 minute | Cook time: 15 minute | Serves 2

1 cup sweet potato mash	minced
½ cup cassava or almond flour	¾ can coconut milk
Olive oil	2 teaspoons tapioca flour
1 sprig parsley diced	2 teaspoons rosemary, diced
Sauce	2 teaspoons Italian oregano, diced
3 tablespoons unsalted butter or ghee	1/3 teaspoon red pepper flakes
1 onion julienned	1 cup spinach or kale
1 teaspoon garlic,	

1. Mix sweet potato mash and flour together until smooth. Roll into 1-inch thick tube and cut into 4 pieces. Stick three in the refrigerator.
2. Cut each segment into 1-inch pieces and stick on baking tray. Drizzle with olive oil and pieces of parsley.
3. Boil pieces until they rise to the top.
4. Transfer gnocchi pieces to skillet and cook over medium heat 1 minute or until each side is a golden brown.
5. In skillet let butter melt them add julienned onions. Turn heat to medium-low and let onions sweat 10 minutes.
6. Whisk in garlic and coconut milk, stirring constantly for 30 seconds. Whisk in tapioca flour, diced rosemary, diced oregano, red pepper flakes.
7. Bring to a low boil for 1-2 minutes constantly stirring.
8. Remove from heat and stir in spinach/kale

Per Serving
Calorie 511| Fats 24.39g| Carbs 118.32g| Protein 10.19g

Paleo Cauliflower Gnocchi with spinach

Prep time: 10 minute | Cook time: 45 minute | Serves 4

5 cups cauliflower, minced	1 teaspoon garlic, minced
1 cup cassava flour	½ teaspoon lemon peel
½ teaspoon smoked paprika	1/3 teaspoon pepper
1 Can coconut milk	2 ½ tablespoons tapioca flour
5 cups spinach or kale	

1. Steam cauliflower 5-7 minutes, ring out water, put in blender along with cassava flour and smoked paprika. Blend until mix is smooth.
2. Roll dough into 1-inch thick tube then cut into four segments, place three in the refrigerator.
3. Cut each segment into 1-inch pieces, drop them into boiling water and let rise to surface.
4. Once they have risen, transfer them to baking tray 20 minutes, turn over, cook another 30 minutes.
5. In skillet over medium-high heat whisk together coconut milk, spinach or kale, minced garlic, lemon peel, pepper, tapioca flour.
6. Stirring continuously until smooth and thickens.
7. Remove from heat and add in spinach or kale and gnocchi.

Per Serving
Calorie 641| Fats 29.3g| Carbs 49.44g| Protein 4.5g

Watermelon Garbanzo & Cucumber Salad

Prep time: 15 minute | Cook time: 0 minute | Serves 6

1 can of garbanzo beans drained and washed (chickpeas)
4 cups chunked watermelon
1 seedless cucumber, sliced
1 cup olive oil
½ teaspoon of red or

white wine vinegar
½ tablespoon rosemary, diced
½ tablespoon Italian oregano, diced
½ tablespoon parsley, diced
2 diced scallions

1. Mix together olive oil, wine vinegar, diced rosemary, diced oregano, diced parsley and diced scallions. Cover and chill.
2. In a large bowl mix together drained and washed garbanzo beans, watermelon chunks, cucumber slices.
3. Pour vinaigrette over salad, toss, serve!

Per Serving

Calorie 687| Fats 45.5g| Carbs 49.44g| Protein 4.5g

Scallion Mushroom Zoodles Salad with Basil

Prep time: 5 minute | Cook time: 0 minute | Serves 4

2 cups zoodles
1 cup scallions, chopped
1 red bell pepper, diced
1 cup sliced mushrooms
2 tablespoons diced Italian oregano
1 ½ tablespoon extra-

virgin olive oil
½ tablespoon balsamic vinegar
2 tablespoons lemon juice
1 tablespoon basil, chopped
1 teaspoon minced garlic

1. Mix together zoodles, chopped scallions, diced red bell pepper, sliced mushrooms, diced Italian oregano,
2. Mix together balsamic vinegar, basil, garlic.

Per Serving

Calorie 151| Fats 9.51g| Carbs 15.96g| Protein 3.35g

Sweet Potato Mango Soup topped with Vinaigrette

Prep time: 10 minute | Cook time: 5 minute | Serves 4

1 medium Sweet Potato
¾ tablespoon Coconut Oil
1 cubed mango
1 cubed avocado
2/3 cup Cucumber, diced
½ tablespoon mint, thinly sliced
½ tablespoon cilantro, diced

½ tablespoon basil, diced
2 tablespoons lime juice
2/3 cup extra virgin olive oil
¼ Teaspoon pepper
1 cup red peppers, julienned
1 sliced jalapeno
1 banana pepper sliced

1. Mix together lime juice, pepper, red peppers, jalapeno slices, banana pepper slices. Cover and chill.
2. Coat sweet potato chunks with coconut oil and cook 2-3 minutes per side to soften. Transfer to plate to cool then put in a bowl along with mango, avocado, cucumber slices, mint, cilantro, basil and stir.
3. Divide between four bowls and top each with vinaigrette.

Per Serving

Calorie 513| Fats 46.6g| Carbs 64.95g| Protein 10.17g

Cheesy red Onions With sautéed Kale

Prep time: 10 minute | Cook time: 5 minute | Serves 2

1 cup kale
1 tablespoon olive oil
½ red onions
¼ Teaspoon salt

2 oz. cheddar cheese
1 garlic clove
¼ Teaspoon dill
2 eggs

1. In a skillet sauté kale until tender
2. In a bowl whisk eggs with salt and cheese
3. In a frying pan heat olive oil and pour egg mixture
4. Add remaining ingredients and mix well
5. When ready serve with sautéed kale

Per Serving

Calorie 514| Fats 38.1g| Carbs 15.91g| Protein 27.1g

Baked Chicken Tenders with Toasted Coconut

Prep time: 10 minute | Cook time: 15 minute | Serves 2

2/3 cup olive oil
½ teaspoon red or white wine
1/3 teaspoon lemon juice
½ teaspoon lemon peel
2 cups zucchini noodles
8 grape organic tomatoes
½ cup toasted

coconut flakes
¼ cup toasted walnuts
8 lemon basil leaves, coarsely chopped
2 teaspoons organic Italian seasoning
6-8 organic chicken tenders
1 teaspoon Mexican seasoning like Tajin
Olive oil for drizzling

1. Preheat oven to 350 and prepare 9x11 dishes.
2. Coat both sides of Chicken tenders with seasoning, lay on tray and drizzle with olive oil, bake 15 minutes, flip and repeat.
3. Mix together olive oil, wine, lemon juice, lemon peel; cover and chill.
4. In bowl combine zoodles, toasted coconut, and toasted walnuts, chopped lemon basil leaves then top with vinaigrette and toss.
5. Divide amongst two plates and serve.

Per Serving
Calorie 945| Fats 85.8g| Carbs 49.44g| Protein 4.5g

Easy No Mayo Apple Cabbage Slaw

Prep time: 5 minute | Cook time: 0 minute | Serves 2

4 cups cabbage
2 cups apples
¼ cup Greek Yogurt

2 tablespoons honey
¼ Teaspoon salt

1. In a bowl mix all ingredients and mix well
2. Serve with dressing

Per Serving
Calorie 351| Fats .94g| Carbs 90.95g| Protein 5.78g

Cauli-Muffins with Italian seasoning

Prep time: 10 minute | Cook time: 30 minute | Serves 12

4 cups cauliflower rice
2 tablespoon extra-virgin olive oil
½ teaspoon garlic, minced
½ teaspoon onion, minced

1 ½ teaspoon Italian seasoning
1 hamburger crumble or 1 ½ cup ground beef, browned and drained

1. Preheat oven to 350 and prepare muffin tin.
2. Mix together cauliflower rice, minced garlic, diced onion, Italian seasoning, ground beef or crumble.
3. Press into muffin tins and bake 30 minutes.
4. Store in airtight container in refrigerator and keep 3-5 days.

Per Serving
Calorie 53| Fats 3.6g| Carbs 36.72g| Protein 9.94g

Crispy Chicken with Sweet Potato & Broccoli Tots

Prep time: 10 minutes | Cook time: 35 minutes | Serves 12

3 oz. chicken patties
1 cup organic breadcrumbs or crushed cornflakes
2 cups sweet potato

mash
2 cups broccoli mash
1 tablespoon paprika
½ tablespoon garlic powder and parsley

1. Preheat oven to 425 and prepare medium sized baking dish.
2. Coat chicken patties with breadcrumbs, spray with olive oil, and bake 35-40 minutes.
3. Blend together sweet potato, broccoli, paprika, garlic powder and parsley.
4. Using hands form into tater tots and fry in coconut oil 2-3 minutes per side.

Per Serving
Calorie 727| Fats 24g| Carbs 49.44g| Protein 4.5g

Coconut Pork chops with Cinnamon sweet potato

Prep time: 10 minutes | Cook time: 10 minutes | Serves 2

1 tablespoon coconut oil
2 thin pork chops
Cinnamon for sprinkling
4 cup sweet potato mash
1 tablespoon chili powder
1 tablespoon paprika
1 tablespoon cayenne pepper
½ tablespoon cumin
½ tablespoon garlic powder and parsley
Coconut oil for frying
Olive oil infused with red pepper

1. In skillet cook pork chops in coconut oil transfer to paper towel lined plates.
2. Mix together sweet potato, chili powder, paprika, cayenne powder, cumin, garlic powder & parsley.
3. With hands form into tater tots and fry in oil 2-3 minutes per side.
4. Before plating, dust both sides of pork chops with cinnamon.

Per Serving

Calorie 230| Fats 11.7g| Carbs 256.5g| Protein 105.3g

Creamy Kidney Beans Curry

Prep time: 10 minute | Cook time: 10 minute | Serves 4

½ Ginger
200 ml cream
5 garlic cloves
5 Tablespoon tomato
puree
2 chilies
2 cans red kidney beans

1. Dice the garlic, ginger and chilli finely
2. Fry them all together
3. After a few minutes, add the tomato puree
4. Pour the cream in mixing slowly
5. Add the kidney beans and season
6. Serve when ready

Per Serving

Calorie 52| Fats 0.24g| Carbs 11.98g| Protein 2.24g

Creamy Peppery Cauliflower with Parsley

Prep time: 5 minutes | Cook time: 10 minutes | Serves 4

1 head of cauliflower, chopped
1/3 cup walnuts
½ cup carrots chopped
1/3 cup cremini mushrooms, sliced
¼ cup onion, minced
1 Teaspoon garlic, minced
4 tablespoons olive oil infused with basil
2 tablespoons cracked black pepper
½ tablespoon parsley, diced

1. In Dutch oven add infused oil and sauté carrots, cremini mushrooms, minced onions, minced garlic.
2. In blender chop cauliflower and walnuts, and then add to Dutch oven.
3. Stir in pepper and parsley.
4. Simmer 7-10 minutes.

Per Serving

Calorie 220| Fats 20.3g| Carbs 38.26g| Protein 14.2g

Broccoli Coconut Cream Soup

Prep time: 15 minute | Cook time: 30 minute | Serves 4

1 (12-ounce) bag frozen broccoli florets, thawed
1 (14-ounce) can cannellini beans, drained and rinsed
1 small onion, peeled
and diced
4 cups Basic Vegetable Stock
1/2 teaspoon ground black pepper
1/2 cup canned full-fat coconut milk

1. Add broccoli, beans, onion, stock, and black pepper to a 2- or 4-quart slow cooker; cover and cook on low for 25 minutes.
2. Use an immersion blender to purée the soup. Stir in coconut milk.
3. Cover and cook for 5 minutes and serve.

Per Serving

Calorie 191| Fats 6g| Carbs 27g| Protein 8g

Baked Vegetables with Lemon Tahini Sauce

Prep time: 5 minute | Cook time: 20 minute | Serves 2

2 cups broccoli trees
2 cups baby carrots
1 cup plum tomatoes, halved
2 cups string beans
Olive oil spray
1 bunch parsley, approx. 1 cup

2 teaspoons lemon juice
2 teaspoons extra virgin olive oil
1 teaspoon garlic, minced
2 tablespoons tahini

1. Preheat oven to 400 and line baking sheet with parchment paper.
2. Layout broccoli trees, baby carrots, halved plum tomatoes and mist with olive oil. Bake 20 minutes.
3. Blend parsley, lemon juice, extra virgin olive oil, minced garlic, and tahini together.
4. Pour sauce over roasted veggie's and enjoy!

Per Serving
Calorie 1202| Fats 107.3g| Carbs 49.65g| Protein 17.13g

Cheesy Ham and Onion scrambled Egg

Prep time: 10 minute | Cook time: 5 minute | Serves 2

8-10 slices ham
1 tablespoon olive oil
½ red onions
¼ Teaspoon salt
2 oz. parmesan

cheese
1 garlic clove
¼ Teaspoon dill
2 eggs

1. In a bowl whisk eggs with salt and parmesan cheese
2. In a frying pan heat olive oil and pour egg mixture
3. Add remaining ingredients and mix well
4. When the ham and eggs are cooked remove from heat and serve.

Per Serving
Calorie 856| Fats 55.74g| Carbs 18.33g| Protein 69.91g

Perfect Broccoli scrambled eggs

Prep time: 10 minute | Cook time: 20 minute | Serves 2

1 cup broccoli
1 tablespoon olive oil
½ red onions
¼ Teaspoon salt

2 oz. cheddar cheese
1 garlic clove
¼ Teaspoon dill
2 eggs

1. In a skillet sauté broccoli until tender
2. In a bowl whisk eggs with salt and cheese.
3. In a frying pan heat olive oil and pour egg mixture.
4. Add remaining ingredients and mix well.
5. When ready serve with sautéed broccoli.

Per Serving
Calorie 515| Fats 38.15g| Carbs 15.65g| Protein 27.68g

Apple Arrowroot and Strawberry Soup

Prep time: 15 minute | Cook time: 15 minute | Serves 4

2 cups water, divided
1/4 cup maple syrup
1 cinnamon stick
11/2 cups unsweetened apple juice
2 cups sliced

strawberries
1 tablespoon lemon juice
1 tablespoon arrowroot powder
1 teaspoon vanilla
1/8 teaspoon salt

1. In a large saucepan, combine 11/2 cups water, maple syrup, cinnamon stick, and apple juice and simmer for 10 minutes. Remove and discard cinnamon.
2. Pour 1 cup of this mixture into a blender or food processor.
3. Add strawberries and purée. Return to saucepan along with lemon juice.
4. Dissolve arrowroot powder in remaining 1/2 cup water and add to pan.
5. Simmer for 4–5 minutes or until thickened. Add vanilla and salt.
6. Cover and chill for 3–4 hours before serving.

Per Serving
Calorie 127| Fats 0g| Carbs 32g| Protein 1g

Celery -Broccoli Macaroni Salad

Prep time: 5 minute | Cook time: 0 minute | Serves 2

2-3 cups cooked macaroni
¼ cup celery
¼ cup broccoli
¼ cup red peppers
¼ cup carrots
Salad dressing

1. In a bowl mix all ingredients and mix well
2. Serve with dressing

Per Serving

Calorie 578| Fats 3.48g| Carbs 113.07g| Protein 21.28g

Easy Tomato Basil and Red Onion Salad

Prep time: 5 minute | Cook time: 0 minute | Serves 2

4 tomatoes
1 red onion
4-5 basil leaves
1 tablespoon olive oil
1 clove garlic
1 cucumber

1. In a bowl mix all ingredients and mix well
2. Serve with dressing

Per Serving

Calorie 281| Fats 14.95g| Carbs 34.81g| Protein 6.99g

Fig and Arugula salad with Blue cheese

Prep time: 5 minute | Cook time: 0 minute | Serves 2

4 figs
½ cup blue cheese
5-6 thin strips prosciutto
4 cups arugula
1 tablespoon olive oil
1 tablespoon balsamic vinegar

1. In a bowl mix all ingredients and mix well
2. Serve with dressing

Per Serving

Calorie 475| Fats 33.74g| Carbs 28.68g| Protein 17.7g

Easy Tasty Tomato Mozzarella Salad

Prep time: 5 minute | Cook time: 0 minute | Serves 2

1 tomato
6 oz. mozzarella
6-7 basil leaves
2 Teaspoon olive oil
1 Teaspoon balsamic vinegar

1. In a bowl mix all ingredients and mix well
2. Serve with dressing

Per Serving

Calorie 347| Fats 9.27g| Carbs 11.73g| Protein 55.13g

Instant Quinoa and Black Bean Salad

Prep time: 5 minute | Cook time: 0 minute | Serves 2

1 can black beans
1 cup cooked quinoa
1 cup corn
1 red bell pepper
1 mango
2 garlic cloves
1 Teaspoon chili powder
2 tablespoons lime juice

1. In a bowl mix all ingredients and mix well
2. Serve with dressing

Per Serving

Calorie 871| Fats 12.08g| Carbs 172.79g| Protein 25.56g

Amazing Olive Pasta and Tomato Salad

Prep time: 5 minute | Cook time: 0 minute | Serves 2

2 tablespoons red wine vinegar
¼ cup olive oil
¼ Teaspoon garlic powder
1 Teaspoon oregano
4 oz. pasta
1 cup olives
½ red onion
1 cucumber
1 cup tomatoes
¼ cup feta cheese

1. In a bowl mix all ingredients and mix well
2. Serve with dressing

Per Serving

Calorie 958| Fats 77.88g| Carbs 58.22g| Protein 12.78g

Garlicky Red Cabbage and Salmon Salad

Prep time: 5 minute | Cook time: 0 minute | Serves 2

2 cooked salmon fillets
1 Teaspoon mustard
1 Teaspoon parsley
1 red onion
2 tablespoons olive oil
¼ Teaspoon garlic powder
½ avocado
1 cup red cabbage

1. In a bowl mix all ingredients and mix well
2. Serve with dressing

Per Serving

Calorie 477| Fats 42.17g| Carbs 26.36g| Protein 4.85g

Chickpea Tomato Fresh Salad with Cucumber

Prep time: 5 minute | Cook time: 0 minute | Serves 2

1 cucumber
1 tomato
1 Can chickpeas
1 tablespoon parsley
1 tablespoon lemon juice
1 cup salad dressing

1. In a bowl mix all ingredients and mix well
2. Serve with dressing

Per Serving

Calorie 1547| Fats 165.3g| Carbs 11.68g| Protein 4.55g

The very best Baby Green Sardine Salad

Prep time: 15 minute | Cook time: 0 minute | Serves 4

1 (4-ounce) can sardines in olive oil, drained
4 cups mixed baby
greens
2 tablespoons olive oil
2 tablespoons lemon juice

1. Place ingredients in a large bowl.
2. Toss to coat and serve immediately.

Per Serving

Calorie 298| Fats 29g| Carbs 4g| Protein 10g

Super Tasty Buttermilk Chicken Salad

Prep time: 5 minute | Cook time: 0 minute | Serves 2

1 cup buttermilk
1 tablespoon mayonnaise
1 Teaspoon salt
1 tablespoon chives
1 Teaspoon garlic
powder
1 Teaspoon parsley
1 Teaspoon basil
1 cup cooked chicken breast

1. In a bowl mix all ingredients and mix well
2. Serve with dressing

Per Serving

Calorie 389| Fats 11.98g| Carbs 14.66g| Protein 53.08g

Avocado Cilantro & Cucumber Soup

Prep time: 15 minute | Cook time: 0 minute | Serves 6

2 medium cucumbers, peeled and diced
1/2 medium red onion, peeled and diced
2 large tomatoes, diced
1/4 cup chopped fresh cilantro
2 avocados, peeled, pitted, and diced
4 cloves garlic, peeled
2 tablespoons lime juice
1 tablespoon apple cider vinegar
3/4 cup Basic Vegetable Stock
1 small jalapeño pepper, seeded and chopped
1 teaspoon salt
1/2 teaspoon ground black pepper

1. In a large bowl, mix together cucumbers, onion, tomatoes, cilantro, and avocados. Set half of the mixture aside.
2. Place the other half in a food processor or blender and pulse to mix.
3. Add garlic, lime juice, vinegar, vegetable stock, and jalapeño and process until smooth.
4. Transfer mixture to the bowl with the reserved cucumbers, onion, tomatoes, cilantro, and avocados. Stir gently to combine.
5. Season with salt and black pepper.
6. Chill in the refrigerator for at least 4 hours before serving.

Per Serving

Calorie 155| Fats 12g| Carbs 14g| Protein 2g

Spicy Pasta with Mackerel and Breadcrumbs

Prep time: 10 minute | Cook time: 10 minute | Serves 4

250 g chard	1 lemon
4 mackerel fillets	30 g breadcrumbs
2 garlic cloves	2 Teaspoon chili
350 g pasta	flakes
3 Tablespoon capers	2 Teaspoon Olive oil

1. Cook the pasta
2. Cook the chard with the pasta for about 5 minutes and drain
3. Squeeze the lemon over and add the zest also
4. Add the capers, a drizzle of oil and chilli flakes
5. Flake the fish over, and mix everything together
6. Serve when ready

Per Serving

Calorie 2272| Fats 44.87g| Carbs 116.28g| Protein 336.83g

Tasty Asparagus Noodles with Soy sauce

Prep time: 10 minute | Cook time: 20 minute | Serves 4

120 g asparagus	2 Tablespoon oil
1 spring onion	5 Tablespoon soy
1 lime	sauce
200 g noodles	30 g maple syrup
250 g tofu	3 Tablespoon sriracha

1. Mix the maple syrup, 3 Tablespoon soy sauce and the sriracha together
2. Cook the noodles
3. Cut the tofu in cubes, then coat in the sriracha mixture
4. Bake at 200C for at least 20 minutes
5. Cut the asparagus and cook with the noodles for about 3 minutes
6. Drain and add ½ lime juice, 2 Tablespoon soy sauce and oil
7. Mix everything together and Serve

Per Serving

Calorie 1529| Fats 92.65g| Carbs 130.7g| Protein 59.77g

Instant Tasty Cheesy Pizza with Tomato sauce

Prep time: 10 minute | Cook time: 15 minute | Serves 8

1 pizza crust	1 cup mozzarella
½ cup tomato sauce	cheese
¼ black pepper	1 cup olives
1 cup pepperoni slices	

1. Spread tomato sauce on the pizza crust
2. Place all the toppings on the pizza crust
3. Bake the pizza at 425 F for 12-15 minutes
4. When ready, remove pizza from the oven and serve

Per Serving

Calorie 641| Fats 29.3g| Carbs 49.44g| Protein 4.5g

Mushroom Coconut Cream Soup

Prep time: 15 minute | Cook time: 30 minute | Serves 4

2 tablespoons olive oil	arrowroot powder
2 tablespoons ghee	2 cups canned full-fat
1 cup finely diced	coconut milk
fresh mushrooms	1/2 teaspoon ground
4 tablespoons	black pepper

1. Heat olive oil and ghee in a deep saucepan over medium heat until sizzling.
2. Add mushrooms and cook until soft, approximately 4–5 minutes.
3. In a medium bowl whisk arrowroot powder into coconut milk. Slowly add to mushrooms. Cook for 5–10 minutes, whisking constantly, until slightly thickened.
4. Carefully pour soup into a greased (coconut oil) 2 1/2-quart slow cooker. Stir in pepper.
5. Cook on high for 15 minutes and serve.

Per Serving

Calorie 333| Fats 32g| Carbs 11g| Protein 3g

Lemony Basil Tomato Vegetable Soup

Prep time: 15 minute | Cook time: 30 minute | Serves 4

5 medium heads garlic, peeled (each clove peeled)	1 large yellow onion, peeled and diced
6 cups Roasted Vegetable	1/4 teaspoon lemon juice
1 (6-ounce) can tomato paste	2 tablespoons olive oil
	2 tablespoons chopped basil

1. Place all ingredients except olive oil and basil into a 4–6-quart slow cooker. Stir.
2. Cover and cook on low for 8 hours or on high for 5 hours.
3. Add olive oil. Use an immersion blender or blend soup in batches in a standard blender until smooth.
4. Garnish with basil and serve.

Per Serving

Calorie 223| Fats 8g| Carbs 37g| Protein 6g

Feel Cool Cucumber Lentil Salad

Prep time: 15 minute | Cook time: 30 minute | Serves 4

1 cup dry green lentils	chopped mint
2 cups water	1/4 cup olive oil
1 cup sliced cucumbers	1/4 cup white balsamic vinegar
3/4 cup sliced strawberries	1/2 orange, juiced
1/2 cup chopped toasted almonds	1 clove garlic, peeled and minced
2 tablespoons	3/4 teaspoon salt
	1/2 teaspoon ground black pepper

1. In a medium pot, combine lentils and water. Bring water to a boil, then reduce heat to a gentle simmer and cook until tender, 20–25 minutes. Drain and let cool.
2. Combine lentils, cucumbers, strawberries, almonds, and mint in a medium bowl and toss to combine.
3. In a small bowl, whisk together remaining ingredients. Pour over lentil mixture and toss to coat.

Per Serving

Calorie 386| Fats 23g| Carbs 35g| Protein 14g

Shallot & Wild Rice with Mushroom Soup

Prep time: 15 minute | Cook time: 30 minute | Serves 4

81/2 cups Roasted Vegetable Stock	11/2 cups thinly sliced leeks
1 cup uncooked wild rice	1/2 cup chopped shallots
3 cups peeled, thinly sliced onions	1 teaspoon maple syrup
2 cups sliced fresh mushrooms	1/2 teaspoon ground black pepper

1. Combine all ingredients in a cooker.
2. Cover and cook on low for 30 minutes.

Per Serving

Calorie 245| Fats 1g| Carbs 54g| Protein 9g

Super Smooth Shallot Zucchini Soup

Prep time: 15 minute | Cook time: 15 minute | Serves 2

3 teaspoons olive oil	edamame, thawed
1/2 cup shredded zucchini	1 cup chopped green onions
1/2 cup chopped shallots	1/2 cup chopped chives
1 clove garlic, peeled and minced	2 cups Basic Vegetable Stock
1 cup frozen shelled	1/2 cup water

1. Heat olive oil in a large soup pot or Dutch oven over medium-low heat. Sauté zucchini, shallots, and garlic in oil for 3–5 minutes.
2. Add edamame, green onions, and chives and cook for 2 minutes more.
3. Add vegetable stock and water. Increase heat to high and bring to a boil. Reduce heat to low and simmer for 5 minutes.
4. In batches, purée soup in a blender or food processor.

Per Serving

Calorie 248| Fats 11g| Carbs 27g| Protein 12g

Classic Five Fruit Salad

Prep time: 15 minute | Cook time: 0 minute | Serves 12

1 large mango, peeled and diced
2 cups fresh blueberries
1 cup sliced bananas
2 cups halved strawberries
2 cups halved seedless grapes
1 cup peeled, sliced nectarines
1/2 cup peeled, sliced kiwi fruit
1/3 cup orange juice
2 tablespoons lemon juice
11/2 tablespoons maple syrup
1/4 teaspoon ground ginger
1/8 teaspoon ground nutmeg

1. In a large bowl, gently toss together mango, blueberries, bananas, strawberries, grapes, nectarines, and kiwi.
2. In a small bowl, stir together orange juice, lemon juice, maple syrup, ginger, and nutmeg; mix well.
3. Chill fruit until needed, for up to 30 minutes.
4. Just before serving, pour orange sauce over fruit and toss gently to coat.

Per Serving
Calorie 90| Fats 1g| Carbs 23g| Protein 1g

Easy Tasty Orange Hazelnuts Salad

Prep time: 15 minute | Cook time: 0 minute | Serves 6

6 large oranges, peeled
3 medium bulbs fennel, finely sliced
1 teaspoon finely chopped hazelnuts
1/3 cup orange juice
2 tablespoons extra-virgin olive oil
1 tablespoon orange zest

1. With a small paring knife, remove each section of the oranges and slice away membrane.
2. Form a mound of sliced fennel on each serving plate and arrange oranges on top. Sprinkle with nuts, then drizzle with orange juice and olive oil.
3. Finish with a sprinkle of zest.

Per Serving
Calorie 170| Fats 5g| Carbs 32g| Protein 3g

Spinach Avocado Salad with Watermelon

Prep time: 15 minute | Cook time: 0 minute | Serves 4

2 large avocados, pitted, peeled, and diced
4 cups cubed watermelon
4 cups fresh baby
spinach leaves
1/2 cup walnut oil
Juice of 1 medium lime
1/2 teaspoon sweet paprika

1. In a medium bowl, combine all ingredients. Mix well and serve.

Per Serving
Calorie 347| Fats 32g| Carbs 17g| Protein 3g

Coconut Leek Soup

Prep time: 15 minute | Cook time: 30 minute | Serves 6

3 tablespoons olive oil
1 medium leek, trimmed and chopped
2 cloves garlic, peeled and minced
4 medium apples, peeled, cored, and chopped
2 tablespoons curry powder
4 cups Basic Vegetable Stock
2 tablespoons lemon juice
1 teaspoon salt
1/8 teaspoon ground white pepper
1 cup canned full-fat coconut milk

1. Heat olive oil in a large saucepan over medium-high heat.
2. Add leek and garlic; cook and stir for 3 minutes.
3. Then add apples; cook and stir for 4 minutes longer.
4. Add curry powder; cook and stir for 2 minutes.
5. Add stock and lemon juice; simmer until apples and leek are very soft, about 20–25 minutes.
6. Purée using an immersion blender, keeping some of the vegetables and fruit whole if you'd like.
7. Season with salt and white pepper.
8. Stir in coconut milk and heat for 1–2 minutes until steaming.
9. Serve immediately.

Per Serving
Calorie 227| Fats 13g| Carbs 27g| Protein 2g

Watermelon Berry & Pine nut Salad

Prep time: 15 minute | Cook time: 30 minute | Serves 4

1 tablespoon hazelnut oil
2 tablespoons olive oil
2 tablespoons lemon juice
2 tablespoons chopped fresh basil leaves
1 tablespoon chopped fresh mint leaves
1/4 teaspoon salt
2 cups sliced strawberries
2 cups blueberries
2 cups cubed watermelon
1/2 cup chopped toasted hazelnuts
1/4 cup toasted pine nuts

1. In a large bowl, combine hazelnut oil, olive oil, lemon juice, basil, mint, and salt and whisk until combined.
2. Add fruits and toss gently until coated.
3. Top with nuts and serve immediately.

Per Serving

Calorie 323| Fats 25g| Carbs 27g| Protein 5g

Spicy Tasty Tahini Date & Carrot Salad

Prep time: 15 minute | Cook time: 0 minute | Serves 4

1/3 cup tahini
1 tablespoon olive oil
2 tablespoons maple syrup
3 tablespoons lemon juice
1/4 teaspoon salt
4 large carrots,
peeled and grated
1/2 cup chopped dates
3 medium clementine, peeled and sectioned
1/3 cup unsweetened coconut flakes

1. In a small bowl, whisk together tahini, olive oil, maple syrup, lemon juice, and salt.
2. Place carrots in a large bowl, and toss well with tahini mixture.
3. Add dates, clementine, and coconut flakes and combine well.
4. Allow to sit for at least 1 hour before serving to soften carrots and dates. Toss again before serving.

Per Serving

Calorie 325| Fats 19g| Carbs 40g| Protein 5g

Rutabaga Turnip Vegetable Salad

Prep time: 15 minute | Cook time: 30 minute | Serves 4

1 large rutabaga, peeled and cubed
1 large turnip, peeled and cubed
6 medium parsnips, peeled and cubed
3 tablespoons olive oil
1 tablespoon
cinnamon
3 cloves garlic, peeled and chopped
1 tablespoon ground ginger
1 teaspoon ground black pepper

1. Preheat oven to 400°F.
2. Place rutabaga, turnip, and parsnips in a large roasting pan and drizzle with olive oil.
3. Sprinkle with cinnamon, garlic, ginger, and black pepper. Toss to coat.
4. Roast for 30 minutes or until toothpick slides through vegetables easily.

Per Serving

Calorie 293| Fats 11g| Carbs 48g| Protein 5g

Lemony Radish Chickpea Salad

Prep time: 15 minute | Cook time: 30 minute | Serves 4

1 (15-ounce) can chickpeas, rinsed and drained
2 cups sliced tomatoes
1 cup chopped, peeled cucumber
1/3 cup seeded, diced yellow bell pepper
1/4 cup sliced radishes
1/4 cup chopped flat-
leaf parsley
1 clove garlic, peeled and finely minced
1 tablespoon lemon juice
3 tablespoons extra-virgin olive oil
1 teaspoon salt
1/2 teaspoon ground black pepper
2 cups torn baby spinach leaves

1. In a large salad bowl, toss chickpeas, tomatoes, cucumber, bell pepper, radishes, and parsley together.
2. Sprinkle garlic, lemon juice, olive oil, salt, and black pepper over salad.
3. Toss to coat. Split spinach among four plates and top with tomato mixture.
4. Serve immediately.

Per Serving

Calorie 248| Fats 13g| Carbs 27g| Protein 8g

Vanilla flavoured Tapioca Blueberry Soup

Prep time: 15 minute | Cook time: 30 minute | Serves 4

3 cups fresh blueberries, divided
2 cups water, divided
1/2 cup freshly squeezed orange juice
2 tablespoons lemon juice

1 cinnamon stick
2 tablespoons honey
1/4 teaspoon salt
2 tablespoons quick-cooking tapioca, ground in a food processor or blender
1 teaspoon vanilla

1. In a large saucepan, combine 2 1/2 cups blueberries, 1 cup water, orange juice, lemon juice, cinnamon stick, honey, and salt. Bring to a simmer over medium heat.
2. Reduce heat to low and simmer for 10 minutes or until blueberries pop.
3. Purée soup in batches in blender or food processor and return to pan.
4. Dissolve tapioca in remaining 1 cup water and add to the soup. Simmer for another 5 minutes until thickened.
5. Cool soup for 25 minutes, and then stir in vanilla. Cover and refrigerate until cold. Stir in remaining 1/2 cup blueberries before serving.

Per Serving
Calorie 128| Fats 0g| Carbs 33g| Protein 1g

Spicy Carrot Root Soup

Prep time: 15 minute | Cook time: 30 minute | Serves 6

1/4 cup olive oil
2 medium onions, peeled and chopped
6 cloves garlic, peeled and minced
1 small butternut squash, peeled, seeded, and cubed
3 large carrots, peeled and sliced
1 medium rutabaga,

peeled and chopped
5 cups Basic Vegetable Stock
1 teaspoon dried marjoram leaves
1 teaspoon dried thyme leaves
1 teaspoon salt
1/4 teaspoon ground black pepper

1. In large soup pot or Dutch oven, heat olive oil over medium heat.

2. Add onions and garlic; cook and stir for 4 minutes.
3. Add squash, carrots, and rutabaga; cook and stir for about 10 minutes or until vegetables start to brown.
4. Add stock, marjoram, thyme, salt, and black pepper and bring to a simmer. Reduce heat to low, cover, and simmer for 25 minutes or until vegetables are tender. Correct seasoning if needed, and serve.

Per Serving
Calorie 205| Fats 10g| Carbs 30g| Protein 3g

Vegan Almond Tomato Soup with cilantro

Prep time: 15 minute | Cook time: 30 minute | Serves 6

2 tablespoons olive oil
2 medium onions, peeled and chopped
2 large red bell peppers, seeded and chopped
4 cloves garlic, peeled and minced
1 (28-ounce) can crushed tomatoes, with liquid

8 cups Roasted Vegetable Stock
1/4 teaspoon ground black pepper
1/4 teaspoon chili powder
2/3 cup natural almond butter
1/2 cup chopped fresh cilantro

1. Heat olive oil in a large skillet over medium-high heat. Cook onions and bell peppers until softened, usually 3–4 minutes.
2. Add garlic and cook for 1 minute more, stirring constantly.
3. Add cooked vegetables to a greased (coconut oil) 6-quart slow cooker.
4. Add tomatoes and their liquid, stock, black pepper, and chili powder to the slow cooker.
5. Cover and cook on high for 20 minutes.
6. One hour prior to serving stir in almond butter. Heat for an additional 45–60 minutes, until soup has been completely warmed through.
7. Garnish with cilantro.

Per Serving
Calorie 366| Fats 21g| Carbs 41g| Protein 11g

Lemony Shrimp & Bell pepper Salad

Prep time: 15 minute | Cook time: 10 minute | Serves 4

1/2 pound large shrimp, peeled and deveined, tails removed
4 medium avocados, peeled, pitted, and diced
1 small sweet onion, peeled and chopped

1 medium red bell pepper, seeded and chopped
1 large ripe tomato, chopped
1/4 cup chopped fresh cilantro
Juice of 1/2 medium lime

1. Bring a medium pot of water to a boil. Add shrimp.
2. Cook for 3–5 minutes until pink and opaque.
3. Drain and place in a medium bowl of ice water to cool, 5 minutes.
4. When cooled, pat dry and cut into bite-sized pieces.
5. Combine shrimp with avocado, onion, bell pepper, tomato, cilantro, and lime juice.
6. Mix well and chill for at least 2 hours before serving.

Per Serving
Calorie 327| Fats 22g| Carbs 22g| Protein 16g

Lemony Lettuce Bell pepper Salad with Fennel

Prep time: 15 minute | Cook time: 5 minute | Serves 4

2 tablespoons olive oil
1/3 cup pine nuts
3 tablespoons sesame seeds
1 medium red bell pepper, seeded and halved
6 romaine lettuce leaves, shredded

1/2 medium bulb fennel, trimmed and diced
1 tablespoon walnut oil
Juice from 1 medium lime
1/2 teaspoon ground black pepper

1. Preheat broiler.
2. In a medium skillet, heat olive oil over medium heat. Sauté pine nuts and sesame seeds for 5 minutes.
3. Grill bell pepper under the broiler until the skin is blackened and the flesh has softened slightly.

4. Place pepper halves in a paper bag to cool slightly. When cool enough to handle, remove skin and slice into strips.
5. Combine red pepper slices, lettuce, and fennel in a large salad bowl.
6. Add walnut oil, lime juice, and black pepper. Mix well to combine. Top with pine nut mixture before serving.

Per Serving
Calorie 309| Fats 28g| Carbs 13g| Protein 5g

Three Beans and Mushroom Salad

Prep time: 15 minute | Cook time: 15 minute | Serves 6

11/2 cups water
1/2 teaspoon salt, divided
1 cup uncooked wild rice
1/4 cup olive oil
3 tablespoons lemon juice
2 tablespoons Dijon mustard
1 tablespoon horseradish
1/8 teaspoon ground black pepper
1 tablespoon chopped fresh dill

1 cup sliced cremini mushrooms
1 cup sliced chanterelle mushrooms
1 cup sliced button mushrooms
1 cup sliced oyster mushrooms
2 cups trimmed green beans
2 cups trimmed wax beans
6 cups mixed salad greens

1. In a small saucepan, bring water and 1/8 teaspoon salt to a boil. Add rice and return to a boil. Reduce the heat to low, cover, and cook for 25 minutes.
2. Turn off the heat and let stand at least 5 minutes. Fluff the rice with a fork.
3. Meanwhile, in a large salad bowl, combine olive oil, lemon juice, mustard, horseradish, remaining salt, pepper, and dill and whisk until combined.
4. Add mushrooms and toss to coat.
5. Steam green beans and wax beans in a large pot over simmering water until tender, about 7–8 minutes. Drain well.
6. Add beans and cooked rice to mushroom mixture and toss to coat.
7. Serve on mixed salad greens.

Per Serving
Calorie 229| Fats 8g| Carbs 30g| Protein 8g

Healthy Sunflower Mushroom Broccoli Salad

Prep time: 15 minute | Cook time: 15 minute | Serves 8

1 large head of broccoli
1 pound green beans, trimmed and cut in half
1 cup frozen shelled edamame, thawed
1 (8-ounce) package mushrooms, sliced
1 medium red bell pepper, seeded and chopped
1 cup chopped walnuts
1/2 cup sunflower seeds
1/4 cup sliced green onions
1/2 cup sliced black olives
1/3 cup olive oil
1/4 cup lemon juice
3 tablespoons grainy mustard
1/2 teaspoon salt
1/8 teaspoon ground black pepper
1/2 cup chopped fresh parsley
2 tablespoons chopped fresh dill

1. Remove florets from broccoli. Peel broccoli stems and slice into 1/2" rounds.
2. Bring a large pot of water to a boil. While water is boiling, prepare large bowl with ice water bath.
3. Add broccoli stems to boiling water; cook for 2 minutes.
4. Add florets and cook for 2–3 minutes more or until tender.
5. Remove with a large strainer and plunge into ice water until cool, 5 minutes.
6. Cook beans in boiling water until crisp-tender, about 4–5 minutes.
7. Remove and plunge into ice water until cool, 5 minutes.
8. Drain cooked vegetables well and place in large serving bowl. Add edamame, mushrooms, bell pepper, walnuts, sunflower seeds, green onions, and olives and toss.
9. In a small bowl, combine olive oil, lemon juice, mustard, salt, and black pepper and mix.
10. Pour over salad and toss to coat. Top with parsley and dill and serve.

Per Serving
Calorie 322| Fats 26g| Carbs 18g| Protein 11g

Super Tasty Spinach Salmon Salad

Prep time: 15 minute | Cook time: 15 minute | Serves 4

4 (4-ounce) salmon fillets
1/2 teaspoon salt, divided
3 cups water
1 bay leaf
1/4 cup extra-virgin olive oil
2 tablespoons lemon juice
1 tablespoon Dijon mustard
1 clove garlic, peeled and minced
1/2 teaspoon dried oregano
1/8 teaspoon ground
black pepper
2 cups chopped curly endive
2 cups chopped butter lettuce
1 cup baby spinach leaves
1 (14-ounce) can plain artichokes, drained and sliced
1 small red onion, peeled and chopped
1 large cucumber, peeled, seeded, and chopped
1/2 cup pitted black olives

1. Arrange salmon in a single layer in a large skillet that is 2" deep.
2. Season with 1/4 teaspoon salt.
3. Add enough water to completely cover the salmon; add bay leaf. Slowly bring water to a simmer.
4. Reduce heat to low, cover the skillet and simmer for 3 to 4 minutes or until the salmon looks opaque. Turn heat off and let stand covered for 10 minutes.
5. Meanwhile in large salad bowl, combine olive oil, lemon juice, mustard, garlic, oregano, remaining salt, and black pepper and mix well.
6. Add endive, lettuce, and spinach and toss to coat.
7. Top with salmon, artichokes, red onion, cucumber, and black olives, toss to coat, and serve.

Per Serving
Calorie 384| Fats 24g| Carbs 17g| Protein 29g

Rosemary Green Beans Millet Salad

Prep time: 15 minute | Cook time: 30 minute | Serves 6

2 cups Basic Vegetable Stock
1 cup dry millet
1 pound fresh green beans, trimmed and cut into 1" pieces
2 teaspoons minced

fresh rosemary
2 teaspoons grated lemon zest
2 tablespoons olive oil
1/2 teaspoon ground black pepper

1. Fill a medium saucepan with stock and bring to a boil over high heat.
2. Add millet, cover, and reduce heat to a simmer.
3. Cook for about 20 minutes, or until stock is absorbed. Remove from heat.
4. Meanwhile, fill a separate medium saucepan with cold salted water and bring to a boil over high heat.
5. Add beans and cook until they are a vibrant green, about 4 minutes.
6. Drain beans and transfer to a large bowl.
7. Add millet and remaining ingredients and toss to coat evenly.
8. Serve warm or at room temperature.

Per Serving
Calorie 193| Fats 6g| Carbs 30g| Protein 5g

Peppery Cauliflower Beets Salad

Prep time: 15 minute | Cook time: 25 minute | Serves 4

4 large beets
1/2 cup water
1/4 cup extra-virgin olive oil
1 medium shallot, minced
2 tablespoons apple cider vinegar
2 tablespoons canned full-fat coconut milk
1 tablespoon maple syrup

1/2 teaspoon salt
1/8 teaspoon ground black pepper
6 cups mixed salad greens
1 medium head cauliflower, broken into florets
1/2 cup toasted pumpkin seeds
1/2 cup sliced fresh basil leaves

1. Preheat oven to 375°F. Place beets in a large baking dish. Add water, cover tightly with foil, and bake for about 25 minutes or until a knife slides easily into a beat.
2. Remove from baking dish and let cool on wire rack.
3. When beets are cool, peel them and cut into 1/2" cubes. Set aside.
4. In a large salad bowl, combine olive oil, shallot, vinegar, coconut milk, maple syrup, salt, and black pepper and mix well. Add greens and toss to coat.
5. Add beets and toss to coat.
6. Top with cauliflower florets, seeds, and basil and serve immediately.

Per Serving
Calorie 323| Fats 22g| Carbs 25g| Protein 10g

CHAPTER 5: DINNER RECIPES

Grilled Salmon & Vegetables Salad
Prep time: 15 minute | Cook time: 0 minute | Serves 2

6 ounces grilled salmon, cut into bite-sized pieces
1 medium zucchini, spiralized with Blade C
1 medium cucumber, peeled and spiralized with Blade C
½ cup celery stalk, chopped
½ cups unsweetened coconut milk
1 small garlic clove, minced
Salt and ground black pepper, as required
2 organic hard-boiled large eggs, peeled and chopped

1. In a large serving bowl, mix together salmon, zucchini, cucumber and celery.
2. In another bowl, add the coconut milk, garlic and seasoning and mix until well combined.
3. Pour the coconut milk mixture over vegetables and gently, toss to coat.
4. Top with chopped eggs and serve.

Per Serving
Calorie 367| Fats 24.9| Carbs 13.7g| Protein 26.6g

Homemade Chicken Carrot Soup
Prep time: 15 minute | Cook time: 20 minute | Serves 4

1 Tablespoon olive oil
½ cup onion, chopped
1 cup carrot, peeled and chopped
2 garlic cloves, minced
2 Tablespoons fresh rosemary, chopped
4½ cups homemade chicken broth
1¼ cups fresh
spinach, torn
1¼ cups grass-fed cooked chicken, shredded
1¼ cups zucchini, spiralized with Blade C
Salt and ground black pepper, as required
2 Tablespoons fresh lemon juice

1. In a large soup pan, heat the oil over medium heat and sauté the onion and carrots for about 8-9 minutes.
2. Add the garlic and rosemary and sauté for about 1 minute.
3. Add the broth and spinach and bring to a boil over high heat.
4. Reduce the heat to medium-low and simmer for about 5 minutes.
5. Add the cooked chicken and zucchini and simmer for about 5 minutes.
6. Stir in the salt, black pepper and lemon juice and remove from heat.
7. Serve hot.

Per Serving
Calorie 174| Fats 6.8| Carbs 8.3g| Protein 19.5g

Beef Sliced with Lemony Arugula
Prep time: 15 minute | Cook time: 10 minute | Serves 4

4 teaspoons fresh lemon juice, divided
1½ Tablespoons extra-virgin olive oil, divided
Salt and ground black pepper, as required
1 pound grass-fed
flank steak, trimmed
Cooking spray, as required
1 teaspoon raw honey
8 cups fresh baby arugula
3 plums, pitted and sliced thinly

1. In a large bowl, place 1 teaspoon of lemon juice, 1½ teaspoons of oil, salt and black pepper and mix well.
2. Add the steak and coat with mixture generously.
3. Grease a nonstick skillet with a little cooking spray and heat over medium-high heat.
4. Add the beef steak and cook for about 5-6 minutes per side.
5. Transfer the steak onto a cutting board and set aside for about 10 minutes before slicing.
6. With a sharp knife, cut the beef steak diagonally across grain in desired size slices.
7. In a large bowl, add the remaining lemon juice, oil, honey, sea salt and black pepper and beat well.
8. Add the arugula and toss well.
9. Divide arugula onto 4 serving plates.
10. Top with beef slices and plum slices evenly and serve.

Per Serving
Calorie 304| Fats 15.1| Carbs 9g| Protein 33g

Tomato Quinoa Carrot Soup

Prep time: 15 minute | Cook time: 30 minute | Serves 6

1 Tablespoon coconut oil
3 carrots, peeled and chopped
3 celery stalks, chopped
1 onion, chopped
4 garlic cloves, minced
4 cups tomatoes, chopped
1 cup red lentils, rinsed and drained
½ cup dried quinoa, rinsed and drained
1½ teaspoons ground cumin
1 teaspoon red chilly powder
5 cups homemade vegetable broth
2 cups fresh spinach, chopped

1. In a large pan, heat the oil over medium heat and sauté the celery, onion and carrot for about 8 minutes.
2. Add the garlic and sauté for about 1 minute.
3. Add the remaining ingredients except spinach and bring to a boil.
4. Reduce the heat to low and simmer, covered for about 20 minutes.
5. Stir in spinach and simmer for about 3-4 minutes.
6. Serve hot.

Per Serving
Calorie 268| Fats 5.1| Carbs 40.2g| Protein 16.4g

Fresh Vegetables and Beef Soup

Prep time: 15 minute | Cook time: 5 minute | Serves 5

1 pound grass-fed beef stew meat, trimmed and cubed
Salt and ground black pepper, as required
2 Tablespoons olive oil, divided
2 medium carrots, peeled and chopped
2 celery stalks, chopped
1 medium onion, chopped
1 cup pumpkin peeled and cube
3 cups fresh tomatoes, chopped finely
4 cups homemade beef broth
1 cup frozen peas, thawed
¼ cup fresh cilantro, chopped

1. Season the beef with a little salt and black pepper evenly.
2. In a large heavy-bottomed pan, heat 1 Tablespoon of oil over medium heat and sear beef for about 4-5 minutes.
3. Transfer the beef into a large bowl and keep aside.
4. In the same pan, heat remaining oil over medium heat and sauté carrot, celery and onion for about 5 minutes.
5. Add the pumpkin and tomatoes and sauté for about 5 minutes.
6. Add the broth and beef and bring to a boil over high heat.
7. Reduce the heat to low and simmer, covered for about 1 hour.
8. Uncover and simmer for about 35 minutes.
9. Stir in the peas, salt and black pepper and simmer for 15 minutes more.
10. Serve hot with the garnishing of cilantro.

Per Serving
Calorie 328| Fats 12.8| Carbs 18.1g| Protein 35.1g

Homemade Pineapple grilled Chicken

Prep time: 15 minute | Cook time: 20 minute | Serves 4

1 (1-inch) piece fresh ginger, minced
2 garlic cloves, minced
1 cup fresh pineapple juice
¼ cup coconut amino
¼ cup extra-virgin olive oil
1 teaspoon ground cinnamon
1 teaspoon ground cumin
Salt, as required
4 grass-fed skinless, boneless chicken breasts

1. In a large Ziploc bag add all ingredients and seal it.
2. Shake the bag to coat the chicken with marinade well.
3. Refrigerate to marinade for about 1 hour.
4. Preheat the grill to medium-high heat. Grease the grill grate.
5. Place the chicken breasts onto the grill and cook for about 10 minutes per side.
6. Serve hot.

Per Serving
Calorie 341| Fats 17.9g| Carbs 12.6g| Protein 32.1g

Super Tasty Peppery Beef with Tomato

Prep time: 15 minute | Cook time: 15 minute | Serves 8

2 Tablespoons extra-virgin olive oil
1 large onion, chopped
1 large green bell pepper, seeded and chopped
4 garlic cloves, minced
1 jalapeño pepper, chopped
1 teaspoon dried thyme, crushed
1 teaspoon dried basil, crushed

2 Tablespoons red chilly powder
1 Tablespoon ground cumin
1 teaspoon ground all spice
2 pounds grass-fed lean ground beef
3 cups fresh tomatoes, chopped finely
2 cups homemade chicken broth
1 cup water

1. In a large pan, heat the oil over medium heat and sauté the onion and bell pepper for about 5-7 minutes.
2. Add garlic, jalapeño pepper, herbs, spices and black pepper and sauté for about 1 minute.
3. Add the beef and cook for about 4-5 minutes.
4. Stir in the tomatoes and cook for about 2 minutes.
5. Add the chicken broth and water and bring to a boil. Reduce the heat to low and simmer, covered for about 25minutes and Serve hot.

Per Serving
Calorie 277| Fats 14.6| Carbs 8g| Protein 25.7g

Rosemary Pepper Chicken with Broccoli Florets

Prep time: 15 minute | Cook time: 30 minute | Serves 6

6 (6-ounce) grass-fed skinless, boneless chicken thighs
3 broccoli heads, cut into florets
4 garlic cloves, minced
¼ cup extra-virgin

olive oil
1 teaspoon dried oregano, crushed
1 teaspoon dried rosemary, crushed
Salt and ground black pepper, as required

1. Preheat the oven to 375 degrees F. Grease a large baking dish.
2. In a large bowl, add all ingredients and toss to coat well.
3. In the bottom of prepared baking dish, arrange the broccoli florets and top with chicken breasts in a single layer.
4. Bake for about 25 minutes.
5. Serve hot.

Per Serving
Calorie 329| Fats 14.9g| Carbs 8.8g| Protein 41.5g

Spicy Chicken with Fresh Cilantro

Prep time: 15 minute | Cook time: 30 minute | Serves 6

4 cups homemade chicken broth, divided
3 cups cooked black beans, divided
1 Tablespoon extra-virgin olive oil
1 large onion, chopped
2 medium poblano peppers, seeded and chopped
1 jalapeño pepper, seeded and chopped
4 garlic cloves, minced

1 teaspoon dried thyme, crushed
1½ Tablespoons ground coriander
1 Tablespoon ground cumin
½ Tablespoon ancho chilly powder
4 cups grass-fed cooked chicken, shredded
1 Tablespoon fresh lime juice
¼ cup fresh cilantro, chopped

1. In a food processor, add 1 cup of broth and 1½ cups of black beans and pulse until smooth.
2. Transfer the beans puree into a bowl and set aside.
3. In a large pan, heat the oil over medium heat and sauté the onion, poblano and jalapeño for about 4-5 minutes.
4. Add the garlic, spices and sea salt and sauté for about 1 minute.
5. Add the beans puree and remaining broth and bring to a boil.
6. Reduce the heat to low and simmer for about 20 minutes.
7. Stir in the remaining beans, chicken and lime juice and bring to a boil.
8. Reduce the heat to low and simmer for about 5-10 minutes.
9. Serve hot with the topping of cilantro.

Per Serving
Calorie 321| Fats 7.4| Carbs 23.7g| Protein 38.3g

Easy Cheddar Chicken Recipe

Prep time: 15 minute | Cook time: 30 minute | Serves 6

4 boneless chicken halves	mix
1 mug cheddar cheese, shredded	2 mugs jarred salsa
4 tbs Taco seasoning	Table salt and black pepper to the taste
	2 tbs sour cream

1. Spray a baking dish with preparing oil, put chicken breasts on it.
2. Season with table salt and pepper and pour salsa all over.
3. Introduce in the oven at 425 degrees F and bake for 30 minutes.
4. Scatter cheese and bake for 5 minutes more.
5. Distribute between plates and serve

Per Serving
Calorie 287| Fats 12.4g| Carbs 6.8g| Protein35.5 g

One Pot Mustard Chicken with Bacon and Onions

Prep time: 15 minute | Cook time: 20 minute | Serves 2

1 Tablespoon olive oil	1/3 mug Dijon mustard
1 and ½ mugs chicken stock	Table salt and black pepper to the taste
3 chicken breasts, skinless and boneless	1 mug yellow onion, sliced off
8 bacon strips, sliced off	¼ tsp. sweet paprika

1. In a pot, consolidate paprika with mustard, table salt and pepper and shake well.
2. Disperse this on chicken bosoms and back rub.
3. Warm up a dish over moderate colossal warmth, embed bacon, shake, plan until it tans and move to a plate.
4. Warm up a similar dish with the oil over moderate massive warmth, embed chicken bosoms, plan for 2 minutes on each side and furthermore move to a plate.
5. Warm up the dish indeed over moderate tremendous warmth, embed stock, shake and bring to a stew.

6. Supplement bacon and onions, table salt and pepper and shake. Return chicken to dish also, shake delicately and stew over moderate warmth for 20 minutes, turning meat midway.
7. Appropriate chicken on plates, sprinkle the sauce over it and serve.

Per Serving
Calorie 762| Fats 52.3g| Carbs 7.11g| Protein65.72 g

Classic Beef-Zucchini Stuffed Bell Peppers

Prep time: 20 minute | Cook time: 30 minute | Serves 5

5 large bell peppers, tops and seeds removed	thyme
1 Tablespoon coconut oil	Salt and ground black pepper, as required
½ large onion, chopped	1 pound grass-fed ground beef
½ teaspoon dried oregano	1 large zucchini, chopped
½ teaspoon dried	3 Tablespoons homemade tomato paste

1. Preheat the oven to 350 degrees F. Grease a small baking dish.
2. In a large pan of the boiling water, place the bell peppers and cook for about 4-5 minutes.
3. Remove from the water and place onto a paper towel, cut side down.
4. Meanwhile, in a large nonstick skillet, melt coconut oil over medium heat and sauté onion for about 3-4 minutes.
5. Add the ground beef, oregano, salt, and pepper and cook for about 8-10 minutes.
6. Add zucchini and cook for about 2-3 minutes.
7. Remove from the heat and drain any juices from the beef mixture.
8. Add the tomato paste and stir to combine.
9. Arrange the bell peppers into the prepared baking dish, cut side upward.
10. Stuff the bell peppers with the beef mixture evenly and bake for 15 minutes. Serve warm.

Per Serving
Calorie 247| Fats 12.1g| Carbs 14.5g| Protein 21.1g

Ground Turkey with fresh Spinach and Tomato

Prep time: 15 minute | Cook time: 30 minute | Serves 6

2 garlic cloves, chopped
2 yellow onions, sliced
1 Tablespoon coriander, ground
2 Tablespoon ginger, grated
1 Tablespoon turmeric
1 Tablespoon cumin, ground
9 ounces turkey

meat, chopped
3 ounces spinach
20 ounces canned tomatoes, sliced off
2 Tablespoon coconut oil
2 Tablespoon coconut cream
Table salt and black pepper to the taste
2 Tablespoon Chilly grinding grains

1. Warm up a dish with the coconut oil over moderate heat, insert onion, shake and prepare for 5 minutes.
2. Insert ginger and garlic, shake and prepare for 1 minute.
3. Insert tomatoes, table salt, pepper, coriander, cumin, turmeric and chilly grinding grains and shake.
4. Insert coconut cream, shake and prepare for 10 minutes.
5. Blend using an immersion blender and combine with spinach and turkey meat.
6. Bring to a simmer, prepare for 15 minute more and serve.

Per Serving
Calorie 1061| Fats 57.5g| Carbs 57.86g| Protein 86.89g

Homemade Turkey Cranberry Salad with Kiwi

Prep time: 15 minute | Cook time: 30 minute | Serves 2

3 kiwis, peeled and sliced
¼ mug cranberries
1 mug cranberry sauce
4 mugs romaine lettuce leaves, torn
¼ mugs turkey breast, prepared and

cubed
1 orange, peeled and slice into small segments
1 red apple, cored and sliced off
3 Tablespoon walnuts, sliced off
1 mug orange juice

1. In a salad pot, combine lettuce with turkey, orange segments, apple pieces, cranberries and walnut and fling to coat.
2. In another pot, combine cranberry sauce and orange juice and shake.
3. Drizzle this over turkey salad, coat and serve with kiwis on top.

Per Servings
Calorie 761| Fats 21.57g| Carbs 27.83g| Protein 112.68g

Spicy Turkey and vegetables Soup

Prep time: 15 minute | Cook time: 30 minute | Serves 6

1 teaspoon olive oil
½ pound cooked ground turkey
½ sweet onion, chopped
1 teaspoon minced garlic
4 cups water
1 cup Easy Chicken Stock
1 celery stalk, chopped
1 carrot, sliced thin
½ cup shredded

green cabbage
½ cup bulgur
2 dried bay leaves
2 Tablespoons chopped fresh parsley
1 teaspoon chopped fresh sage
1 teaspoon chopped fresh thyme
Pinch red pepper flakes
Freshly ground black pepper

1. Place a large saucepan over medium-high heat and add the olive oil. Sauté the turkey for about 5 minutes or until the meat is cooked through.
2. Add the onion and garlic and sauté for about 3 minutes or until the vegetables are softened.
3. Add the water, chicken stock, celery, carrot, cabbage, bulgur, and bay leaves.
4. Bring the soup to a boil and then reduce the heat to low and simmer for about 25 minutes or until the bulgur and vegetables are tender.
5. Remove the bay leaves and stir in the parsley, sage, thyme, and red pepper flakes.
6. Season with pepper and serve.

Per Serving
Calorie 777| Fats 33.09g| Carbs 49.08g| Protein74.77 g

Grandma's Grilled Peanut Butter Chicken

Prep time: 15 minute | Cook time: 10 minute | Serves 6

A pinch of red pepper flakes
Table salt and black pepper to the taste
½ tsp. ginger, ground
1/3 mug peanut butter
2 and ½ pounds

chicken
1 Tablespoon coconut amino
1 Tablespoon apple cider vinegar
1 garlic clove, chopped
½ mug warm water

1. In blender combine peanut butter with water, amino, table salt, pepper, pepper flakes, ginger, garlic and vinegar and blend well.
2. Pat dry chicken pieces organize them in a dish and pour the peanut butter marinade over it.
3. Fling to coat and keep in the fridge for 1 hour.
4. Put chicken pieces skin side down on your preheated grill over moderate immense heat, prepare for 10 minutes, flip, brush with some of the marinades and prepare them for 10 minutes more.
5. Distribute between plates and serve.

Per Serving
Calorie 778| Fats 41.96g| Carbs 10.88g| Protein 84.13g

Oven cooked Chicken with bacon Asiago cheese

Prep time: 15 minute | Cook time: 10 minute | Serves 2

½ mug avocado oil
1 egg, whisked
Table salt and black pepper to the taste
1 mug asiago cheese, shredded
4 bacon slices, prepared and

crumbled
1 ½ chicken breasts, skinless and boneless
1 Tablespoon water
¼ tsp. garlic grinding grains
1 mug parmesan cheese, grated

1. In a pot, combine parmesan cheese with garlic, table salt and pepper and shake. Put whisked egg in another pot and combine with the water.

2. Season chicken with table salt and pepper and dip each piece into egg and then into cheese combine.
3. Warm up a dish with the oil over moderate immense heat, insert chicken breasts, prepare until they are golden on both sides and shift to a baking dish.
4. Introduce in the oven at 350 degrees F and bake for 20 minutes.
5. Top chicken with bacon and asiago cheese, introduce in the oven, turn on broiler and broil for a couple of minutes.
6. Serve warm.

Per Serving
Calorie 1481| Fats 105.54g| Carbs 14.94g| Protein 115.65g

Muenster -Bacon Stuffed Chicken Breast

Prep time: 15 minute | Cook time: 30 minute | Serves 6

4 ounces cheddar cheese, cubed
2 ounces provolone cheese, cubed
1 zucchini, shredded
½ pounds chicken breasts
2 ounces Muenster cheese, cubed

2 ounces cream cheese
Table salt and black pepper to the taste
1 tsp. garlic, chopped
½ mug bacon, prepared and crumbled

1. Season zucchini with table salt and pepper, leave aside few minutes, press well and shift to a pot.
2. Insert bacon, garlic, a lot of table salt and pepper, cream cheese, cheddar cheese, Muenster cheese and provolone cheese and shake.
3. Slice slits into chicken breasts, season with table salt and pepper and stuff with zucchini and cheese mix.
4. Put on a lined baking sheet, introduce within the oven at 400 degrees F and bake for forty-five minutes.
5. Distribute between plates and serve.

Per Serving
Calorie 1189| Fats 79.54g| Carbs 21.5g| Protein 95.67g

Lemony Sole Fry with Chopped Scallions

Prep time: 15 minute | Cook time: 10 minute | Serves 6

¼ cup all-purpose flour
¼ teaspoons freshly ground black pepper
12 ounces sole fillets, deboned and skinned
2 Tablespoons olive oil
1 scallion, both green and white parts, chopped
Lemon wedges, for garnish

1. In a large plastic freezer bag, shake together the flour and pepper to combine.
2. Add the fish fillets to the flour and shake to coat.
3. In a large skillet over medium-high heat, heat the olive oil.
4. When the oil is hot, add the fish fillets and fry for about 10 minutes, turning once, or until they are golden and cooked through.
5. Remove the fish from the oil onto paper towels to drain.
6. Serve topped with chopped scallions and a squeeze of lemon

Per Serving
Calorie 1678| Fats 106.2 g| Carbs 57.82 g| Protein 121.85g

Peppery Beef Roast with gravy

Prep time: 15 minute | Cook time: 30 minute | Serves 6

1-pound boneless beef chuck or rump roast
½ teaspoons freshly ground black pepper
1 Tablespoon olive oil
½ small, sweet onion, chopped
2 teaspoons minced garlic
1 teaspoon dried thyme
1 cup plus 3 Tablespoons water
2 Tablespoons cornstarch

1. Place a large stockpot over medium heat.
2. Season the roast with pepper.
3. Add the oil to the stockpot and brown the meat all over.
4. Remove the meat to a plate; set aside.
5. Sauté the onion and garlic in the stockpot for about 3 minutes or until they are softened.
6. Return the beef to the pot with any accumulated juices and add the thyme and 1 cup water.
7. Bring the liquid to a boil and then reduce the heat to low
8. Cover and simmer for about 25 minutes or until the beef is very tender.
9. In a small bowl, stir together the cornstarch and 3 Tablespoons water to form slurry.
10. Whisk the slurry into the liquid in the pot and cook for 5 minutes to thicken the sauce and Serve the roast with the gravy.

Per Serving
Calorie 1034| Fats 51.96g| Carbs 19.92g| Protein 121.71 g

Cilantro Coconut Chicken Tenders

Prep time: 15 minute | Cook time: 15 minute | Serves 6

3 Tablespoons olive oil, divided
6 boneless, skinless chicken thighs
1 small, sweet onion
2 teaspoons minced garlic
1 teaspoon grated
fresh ginger
1 Tablespoon Hot Curry Powder
¾ cup water
¼ cup coconut milk
2 Tablespoons chopped fresh cilantro

1. In a large skillet over a medium-high heat, heat 2 Tablespoons of the oil.
2. Add the chicken and cook for about 10 minutes
3. With tongs, remove the chicken to a plate and set aside.
4. Add the remaining 1 Tablespoon of oil to the skillet and sauté the onion, garlic, and ginger for about 3 minutes or until they are softened.
5. Stir in the curry powder, water, and coconut milk.
6. Return the chicken to the skillet and bring the liquid to a boil.
7. Reduce the heat to low, cover the skillet, and simmer for about 25 minutes or until the chicken is tender and the sauce is thick.
8. Serve topped with cilantro.

Per Serving
Calorie 633| Fats 56g| Carbs 34.11g| Protein 5.36g

Creamy Garlic Mushroom Chicken

Prep time: 15 minute | Cook time: 20 minute | Serves 6

1 mug coconut milk
1 yellow onion, sliced off
1-pound chicken breasts, slice into moderate pieces
1 and ½ teaspoons thyme, dried
2 Tablespoon parsley, sliced off
4 garlic cloves, chopped
8 ounces mushrooms, roughly sliced off
¼ tsp. celery seeds, ground
1 mug chicken stock
Table salt and black pepper to taste
4 Zucchinis, slice with a spiralized

1. Put chicken in your slow preparer. Insert table salt, pepper, onion, garlic, mushrooms, coconut milk, celery seeds, stock, parsley and thyme.
2. Unwrap up pot; insert a lot of table salt and pepper if required and the rest of the parsley and shake.
3. Warm up a dish with water over moderate heat, insert some table salt, bring to a boil, insert zucchini pasta, and prepare for 15 minute and drain.
4. Distribute on plates, insert chicken combine on prime and serve.

Per Serving
Calorie 863| Fats 43.05g| Carbs 14.52g| Protein 103.23g

Creamy Pepper Chicken with Onion

Prep time: 15 minute | Cook time: 15 minute | Serves 2

1 chicken breast, skinless and boneless
Table salt and black pepper to the taste
2 Tablespoon ghee
1 green onion, sliced off
8 ounces sour cream

1. Warm up a dish with the ghee over moderate immense heat, insert chicken items, season with table salt and pepper, wrap up, reduce heat and simmer for 10 minutes.
2. Unwrap up dish, turn chicken items and prepare them Wrap upped for 10 minutes additional.

3. Insert inexperienced onions, shake and prepare for 2 minutes.
4. Remove heat, insert additional table salt and pepper if required, insert sour cream, shake well, wrap up dish and leave aside for 5 minutes.
5. Shake once more, distribute between plates and serve.

Per Serving
Calorie 825| Fats 50.96g| Carbs 20.36g| Protein 69.3g

Fresh Peas with Ground Beef and Almonds

Prep time: 15 minute | Cook time: 30 minute | Serves 6

2 Tablespoons olive oil
1 pound grass-fed lean ground beef
1 large onion, chopped finely
2 garlic cloves, minced
½ Tablespoon fresh ginger, minced
1 teaspoon ground coriander
1 teaspoon ground
cumin
¼ teaspoon chili powder
2 medium tomatoes, seeded and chopped
½ cup homemade chicken broth
Salt and ground black pepper, as required
2¼ cups fresh peas, shelled
2 Tablespoons fresh cilantro, chopped

1. In a large skillet, heat the oil over medium heat and cook the beef for about 4-5 minutes or until browned completely.
2. With a slotted spoon, transfer the beef into a large bowl.
3. In the same skillet, add onion and sauté for about 4-6 minutes.
4. Add the garlic, ginger, coriander, cumin and chilly powder and sauté for about 1 minute.
5. Add the tomatoes and cook for about 2-3 minutes, crushing completely with the back of spoon.
6. Stir in the beef and broth and bring to a boil.
7. Reduce the heat to medium-low and simmer, covered for about 8-10 minutes, stirring occasionally.
8. Stir in peas and cook for 10-15 minutes.
9. Remove from heat and serve hot with the garnishing of almonds and cilantro leaves.

Per Serving
Calorie 243| Fats 11.9g| Carbs 12.7g| Protein 19.5g

Chicken stuffed with Cream cheese & Spinach

Prep time: 15 minute | Cook time: 15 minute | Serves 2

4 ounces cream cheese, soft	prepared and sliced off
3 ounces feta cheese, crumbled	1 chicken breast
1 garlic clove, chopped	Table salt and black pepper to the taste
8 ounces spinach,	1 Tablespoon coconut oil

1. In a pot, combine feta cheese with cream cheese, spinach, table salt, pepper and therefore the garlic and shake well.
2. Put chicken breasts on a working surface, slice a pocket in each, stuff them with the spinach combine and season them with table salt and pepper to the taste.
3. Warm up a dish with the oil over moderate immense heat, insert stuffed chicken, prepare for 5 minutes on every side and then introduce everything within the oven at 450 degrees F.
4. Bake for 10 minutes, distribute between plates and serve.

Per Serving
Calorie 1250| Fats 91.96g| Carbs 20.93g| Protein 88.19g

Sweet and Spicy Orange Chicken

Prep time: 10 minute | Cook time: 20 minute | Serves 6

3 garlic cloves, minced	blossom water
½ cup fresh orange juice	¼ teaspoon ground ginger
1 Tablespoon apple cider vinegar	¼ teaspoon ground cinnamon
2 Tablespoons coconut amino	Salt, as required
½ teaspoon orange	2 pounds grass-fed skinless, bone-in chicken thighs

1. For marinade, in a large bowl, place all ingredients except chicken and mix well.
2. Add the chicken and coat with marinade generously.
3. Cover the bowl of chicken and refrigerate for about 2 hours.

4. Remove the chicken from bowl, reserving marinade.
5. Heat a large nonstick wok, over medium-high heat and cook the chicken for about 5-6 minutes or until golden brown.
6. Flip the side and cook for about 4 minutes.
7. Add the reserved marinade and bring to a boil.
8. Now, reduce the heat to medium-low heat and cook, covered for about 6-8 minutes or until sauce becomes thick.
9. Serve hot.

Per Serving
Calorie 305| Fats 11.3g| Carbs 8.3g| Protein 44g

Hot & Spicy Pineapple Coconut Chicken

Prep time: 20 minute | Cook time: 25 minute | Serves 5

1 Tablespoon extra-virgin olive oil	pepper, seeded and chopped
1 large onion, chopped	1 medium green bell pepper, seeded and chopped
1 garlic clove, minced	1 medium orange bell pepper, seeded and chopped
1 teaspoon fresh ginger, minced	
2 grass-fed skinless, boneless chicken breasts, cubed	2 Tablespoons coconut amino
2 cups fresh pineapple, cubed	1 Tablespoon apple cider vinegar
2 tomatoes, seeded and chopped	Ground black pepper, as required
1 medium red bell	

1. In a large skillet, heat oil over medium heat.
2. Add onion and sauté for about 4-5 minutes.
3. Add garlic and ginger and sauté for about 1 minute.
4. Add chicken and cook for about 10 minutes or until browned from all sides.
5. Add pineapple, tomatoes and bell peppers and cook for about 5-6 minutes or until vegetables become tender.
6. Add the coconut amino, vinegar and pepper and cook for about 2-3 minutes.
7. Serve hot.

Per Serving
Calorie 194| Fats 5.6g| Carbs 20.5g| Protein 17.1g

Nutty Fruity Chicken Zucchini Noodles

Prep time: 15 minute | Cook time: 15 minute | Serves 3

2 zucchinis, spiralized with Blade C
Salt, as required
1½ teaspoons olive oil
½ teaspoon fresh ginger, minced
¾ cup rhubarb, chopped
10 ounces grass-fed skinless, boneless chicken breasts, cubed
4 teaspoons raw honey
1 teaspoon fresh lime zest, grated finely
¼ cup plus 2 teaspoons fresh orange juice, divided
1 Tablespoon fresh lime juice
2 teaspoons fresh mint leaves, minced
½ cup fresh strawberries, hulled and sliced
2 Tablespoons almonds, toasted and slivered

1. Arrange a large strainer over the sink.
2. Place the zucchini noodles in a strainer and sprinkle with a pinch of salt.
3. Set aside to release the excess moisture.
4. In a large skillet, heat the oil over medium heat and cook the ginger and rhubarb for about 2-3 minutes.
5. Stir in the chicken cubes and cook for about 4-5 minutes.
6. Add the honey, lime zest, ¼ cup of orange juice, lime juice and a pinch of salt and stir to combine.
7. Now, increase the heat to high and bring to a boil.
8. Now, reduce the heat to medium and simmer for about 4-5 minutes, stirring occasionally.
9. Remove from the heat.
10. Meanwhile, squeeze the moisture from zucchini and pat dry with paper towels.
11. In a small bowl, place the remaining orange juice and mint and mix.
12. Divide the zucchini noodles in serving plates and drizzle with mint mixture.
13. Place the chicken mixture, strawberries and almonds over zucchini noodles and gently stir to combine.
14. Serve immediately.

Per Serving
Calorie 236| Fats 8.1g| Carbs 18.8g| Protein 24.2g

Apple Glazed Roasted Turkey Breast

Prep time: 20 minute | Cook time: 30 minute | Serves 3

For Turkey Rub:
1 (5-pound) whole, bone-in turkey breast
2 Tablespoons fresh thyme leaves, chopped
2 Tablespoons fresh rosemary, chopped
2 Tablespoons olive oil

For Stuffing:
1 small onion, thinly sliced
1 apple, peeled and thinly sliced
1 pear, peeled and thinly sliced
¼ cup dried cranberries

For Glaze:
2 cups fresh apple juice, divided
1 Tablespoon olive oil
1 Tablespoon brown
mustard
½ Tablespoon coconut sugar

1. Preheat the oven to 325 degrees F. Arrange a rack in a roasting pan.
2. Arrange turkey breast into the prepared roasting pan, skin-side up.
3. With your fingers, gently loosen the skin from the meat, making deep pockets between the skin and meat.
4. For rub: in a small bowl, mix together fresh herbs and oil.
5. Rub half of herb mixture on the meat and then, spread the remaining paste evenly over the top of the skin.
6. For stuffing: in a bowl, mix together all ingredients.
7. Stuff each pocket with the stuffing mixture.
8. In the bottom of roasting pan, pour 1 cup of apple juice.
9. Roast for about 30 minute. (If skin becomes brown during roasting, then cover the pan with a piece of foil).
10. Meanwhile, for glaze: in a pan, add remaining apple juice, oil, mustard and brown sugar and bring to a boil.
11. Reduce the heat and simmer until thick glaze is formed.
12. In the last 5 minutes of cooking, coat turkey breast with glaze evenly.
13. Remove from oven and cut turkey into desired slices before serving.

Per Serving
Calorie 290| Fats 9.2g| Carbs 19.1g| Protein 32.5g

Garlic Lamb with Kidney Beans

Prep time: 15 minute | Cook time: 30 minute | Serves 6

1½ Tablespoons extra-virgin olive oil, divided
1 cup onion, chopped
6 large garlic cloves, minced
2 dried New Mexico chiles, stemmed, seeded and torn
3 dried ancho chiles, stemmed, seeded and torn
2 teaspoons dried oregano, crushed
1½ teaspoons ground cumin
2 large plum tomatoes, chopped
2 cups homemade chicken broth
1 pound grass-fed lamb stew meat, trimmed and cubed
Salt and ground black pepper, as required
15 ounces cooked kidney beans

1. In an oven-proof pan, heat 1 Tablespoon of oil over medium heat and sauté the onion for about 4-5 minutes.
2. Add the garlic, both chiles and spices and sauté for about 1 minute.
3. Add the tomatoes and broth and bring to a boil.
4. Reduce the heat to medium-low and simmer, covered for about 10 minutes.
5. Preheat the oven to 325 degrees F. Arrange a rack in the center of the oven.
6. Remove the pan from heat and set aside to cool slightly.
7. Transfer the Chile mixture into a blender and pulse until pureed.
8. Return the puree in the same pan.
9. Meanwhile, in another pan, heat the remaining oil over medium-high heat and cook the lamb with salt and black pepper k for about 3-4 minutes.
10. Transfer the cooked lamb in the pan with puree and stir to combine.
11. Cover the pan and bake for about 30 minutes.
12. Remove pan from the oven and place over medium-low heat.
13. Simmer, uncovered for about 5 minutes.
14. Stir in kidney beans and simmer for about 5 minutes.
15. Serve hot.

Per Serving
Calorie 430| Fats 8.3| Carbs 49.7g| Protein 40g

Sweet and spicy Arrowroot Flank Steak

Prep time: 15 minute | Cook time: 12 minute | Serves 4

2 Tablespoons arrowroot flour
Salt and ground black pepper, as required
1 pound grass-fed flank steak, cut into ¼-inch thick slices
½ cup plus 1 Tablespoon coconut oil, divided
2 garlic cloves, minced
1 teaspoon ground ginger
Pinch of red pepper flakes, crushed
1/3 cup raw honey
½ cup homemade beef broth
½ cup coconut amino
3 scallions, chopped

1. In a bowl, add the arrowroot flour, salt and black pepper and mix well.
2. Coat the beef slices with arrowroot flour mixture evenly.
3. Shake off the excess arrowroot flour mixture and set aside for about 10-15 minutes.
4. For sauce: in a pan, melt 1 Tablespoon of coconut oil over medium heat and sauté the garlic, ginger powder and red pepper flakes for about 1 minute.
5. Add the honey, broth and coconut amino and stir to combine well.
6. Now, increase the heat to high and cook for about 3 minutes, stirring continuously.
7. Remove from the heat and set aside.
8. In a large skillet, melt the remaining coconut oil over medium heat and stir fry the beef for about 2-3 minutes.
9. Remove the oil from skillet and stir fry for about 1 minute.
10. Stir in the honey sauce and cook for about 3 minutes.
11. Stir in the scallion and cook for about 1 minute more.
12. Serve hot.

Per Serving
Calorie 586| Fats 36.9g| Carbs 31.6g| Protein 32.8g

Beef Cauliflower stir fry with Cilantro leaves

Prep time: 15 minute | Cook time: 12 minute | Serves 4

1 Tablespoon coconut oil	3½ cups cauliflower florets
4 garlic cloves, minced	3 Tablespoons coconut amino
1 pound grass-fed beef sirloin steak, cut into bite-sized pieces	¼ cup fresh cilantro leaves, chopped

1. In a large skillet, heat the oil over medium heat and sauté the garlic for about 1 minute.
2. Add beef and stir to combine.
3. Increase the heat to medium-high and cook for about 6-8 minutes or until browned from all sides.
4. Meanwhile, in a pan of boiling filtered water, add cauliflower and cook for about 5-6 minutes.
5. Drain the cauliflower completely.
6. Add the cauliflower and coconut amino in skillet with beef and cook for about 2-3 minutes.
7. Serve with the garnishing of cilantro.

Per Serving
Calorie 278| Fats 10.6g| Carbs 7.9g| Protein 36.3g

Beef Bowl with Plum Tomato and Lentils

Prep time: 15 minute | Cook time: 30 minute | Serves 6

3 Tablespoons extra-virgin olive oil, divided	2 cups homemade chicken broth
1 onion, chopped	2 teaspoons cumin seeds
1 Tablespoon fresh ginger, minced	½ teaspoon cayenne pepper
4 garlic cloves, minced	1 pound grass-fed lean ground beef
3 plum tomatoes, chopped finely	1 jalapeño pepper, seeded and chopped
2 cups dried red lentils, soaked for 30 minutes and drained	2 scallions, chopped

1. In a Dutch oven, heat 1 Tablespoon of oil over medium heat and sauté the onion, ginger and garlic for about 5 minutes.
2. Stir in the tomatoes, lentils and broth and bring to a boil
3. Reduce the heat to medium-low and simmer, covered for about 30 minutes.
4. Meanwhile, in a skillet, heat remaining oil over medium heat.
5. Add the cumin seeds and sauté for about 30 seconds.
6. Add the paprika and sauté for about 30 seconds.
7. Transfer the mixture into a small bowl and set aside.
8. In the same skillet, add the beef and cook for about 4-5 minutes.
9. Add jalapeño and scallion and cook for about 4-5 minutes.
10. Add the spiced oil mixture and stir to combine well.
11. Transfer the beef mixture into the simmering lentils and simmer for about 10-15 minutes or until desired doneness.
12. Serve hot.

Per Serving
Calorie 469| Fats 13.3g| Carbs 45.1g| Protein 42.3g

Instant Parmesan Halibut

Prep time: 15 minute | Cook time: 25 minute | Serves 2

2 Tablespoon green onions, sliced off	½ mug parmesan, grated
6 garlic cloves, chopped	¼ mug ghee
A dash of Tabasco sauce	¼ mug mayonnaise
4 halibut fillets	Table salt and black pepper to the taste
	Juice of ½ lemons

1. Season halibut with table salt, pepper and some of the lemon juice
2. Place in a very baking dish and prepare in the oven at 450 degrees F for 6 minutes.
3. Meanwhile, warm up a dish with the ghee over moderate heat, insert parmesan, mayo, inexperienced onions, Tabasco sauce, garlic and the rest of the lemon juice and shake well.
4. Take fish out of the oven, drizzle parmesan sauce all over, flip oven to broil and broil your fish for three minutes.
5. Distribute between plates and serve.

Per Serving
Calorie 1118| Fats 63.85g| Carbs 55.21g| Protein 82.62g

Creamy Mushroom Pepper curry soup

Prep time: 5 minute | Cook time: 10 minute | Serves 4

3 ½ cups of baby bella mushrooms 1 8 oz package, chopped
½ cup yellow onion diced
2 cloves garlic diced
2 thyme sprigs just leaves
Salt and pepper to taste
½ cup raw cashews or

place in hot/boiling water for 15+ minutes until soft, soaked for 2 hours
2 cups chicken or veggie stock
1 Tablespoon extra virgin olive oil
1 Tablespoons of butter or olive oil

1. Heat a skillet over medium high heat, add butter or olive.
2. Add garlic, onions, thyme leaves, salt and pepper and cook until onions are translucent and fragrant.
3. Add mushrooms and continue to cook until mushrooms are soft and the moisture from them has evaporated off, about 5-6 minutes.
4. Drain the cashews and place them in a high speed blender.
5. Add the chicken or veggie stock and blend on high until mixture is silky and smooth.
6. Next add ½ of the mushroom onion mixture and blend until smooth.
7. Pour into a serving bowl and mix in the remaining mushroom and onion mixture.
8. Serve and Enjoy!

Per Serving
Calorie 525| Fats 31.24g| Carbs 43.49g| Protein 19.72g

Homemade Lemon and Garlic Salmon

Prep time: 15 minute | Cook time: 25 minute | Serves 6

1 Tablespoon Italian seasoning
2 Tablespoon capers
3 Tablespoon lemon juice
4 garlic cloves,

chopped
3 salmon fillets
Table salt and black pepper to the taste
1 Tablespoon olive oil
2 Tablespoon ghee

1. Warm up a dish with the olive oil over moderate heat.

2. Insert fish fillets skin side up.
3. Season them with table salt, pepper and Italian seasoning.
4. Prepare for 2 minutes, flip and prepare for 2 additional minutes, take away heat.
5. Finish off dish and leave aside for 15 minutes.
6. Shift fish to a plate and leave them aside.
7. Warm up the same dish over moderate heat, insert capers, lemon juice and garlic, shake and prepare for two minutes.
8. Take the dish off the warmth, insert ghee and shake terribly well.
9. Return fish to dish and fling to coat with the sauce.
10. Distribute between plates and serve.

Per Serving
Calorie 197| Fats 13.91g| Carbs 17.21g| Protein 2.62g

Baked Chicken with Mozzarella & Tomato

Prep time: 15 minute | Cook time: 30 minute | Serves 3

1 chicken breast, skinless and boneless and sliced
1 tomato, sliced off
½ tsp. oregano, dried
½ tsp. basil, dried
1 zucchini, sliced off
Table salt and black

pepper to the taste
1 tsp. garlic grinding grains
1 Tablespoon avocado oil
½ mug mozzarella cheese, shredded

1. Season chicken with table salt, pepper and garlic grinding grains. Warm up a dish with the oil over moderate heat, insert chicken slices, brown on all sides and shift them to a baking dish.
2. Warm up the dish again over moderate heat, insert zucchini, oregano, tomato, basil, table salt and pepper, shake, prepare for two minutes and pour over chicken.
3. Introduce within the oven at 325 degrees F and bake for 20 minutes. Scatter mozzarella over chicken, introduce in the oven once more and bake for five minutes more.
4. Distribute between plates and serve.

Per Serving
Calorie 652| Fats 41.04g| Carbs 6.64g| Protein 62.11g

One pot Chicken with Guar Parsley and Sauce

Prep time: 15 minute | Cook time: 30 minute | Serves 2

Table salt and black pepper to the taste	½ chicken breast
2 Tablespoon coconut oil	½ tsp. onion grinding grains
1 tsp. Italian seasoning	½ tsp. garlic grinding grains
½ mugs chicken stock	2 teaspoons guar parsley, sliced

1. Rub chicken with oil, garlic grinding grains, table salt, pepper, Italian seasoning and onion grinding grains.
2. Put the remainder of the oil into an immediate pot and add chicken.
3. Insert stock, conclude pot and prepare on Immense for 20 minutes. Shift chicken to a platter and leave aside for now.
4. Set the moment pot on Sauté mode, insert guar parsley, sliced, shake and prepare until it thickens.
5. Pour sauce over chicken and serve.

Per Serving
Calorie 847| Fats 40.33g| Carbs 19.06g| Protein 99.49g

Baked Ricotta Chicken

Prep time: 15 minute | Cook time: 30 minute | Serves 6

2 teaspoons Italian seasoning	2 Tablespoon parsley, sliced off
Table salt and black pepper to the taste	4 garlic cloves, chopped
½ mug ricotta cheese	2 teaspoons onion grinding grains
1 mug parmesan, grated	2 teaspoons chives, sliced off
1 mug mozzarella, shredded	2 Tablespoon parsley, sliced off
1 mug marinara sauce	1 garlic clove, chopped
1 pound chicken meat, ground	

1. In a pot, join chicken with half of the marinara sauce, table salt, pepper, Italian flavoring, 4 garlic cloves, onion granulating grains and 2 Tablespoon parsley and shake well.

2. In another pot, consolidate ricotta with half of the parmesan, half of the mozzarella, chives, 1 garlic clove, table salt, pepper and 2 Tablespoon parsley and shake well.
3. Put half of the chickens consolidate into a portion dish and Scatter equally. Addition cheddar filling and furthermore Scatter.
4. Top with the remainder meat and Scatter once more.
5. Present meatloaf in the broiler at 400 degrees F and prepare for 20 minutes.
6. Remove meatloaf from the broiler, Scatter the remainder of the marinara sauce, the remainder of the parmesan and mozzarella and heat for 10 minutes more.
7. Leave meatloaf to chill off, cut, disseminate among plates and serve.

Per Serving
Calorie 1148| Fats 37.66g| Carbs 67.51g| Protein 133.1g

Baked Lemon Haddock

Prep time: 20 minute | Cook time: 20 minute | Serves 2

½ cup breadcrumbs	¼ teaspoons freshly ground black pepper
3 Tablespoons chopped fresh parsley	1 Tablespoon melted unsalted butter
1 Tablespoon lemon zest	12-ounces haddock fillets, deboned and skinned
1 teaspoon chopped fresh thyme	

1. Preheat the oven to 350°F.
2. In a small bowl, stir together the breadcrumbs, parsley, lemon zest, thyme, and pepper until well combined.
3. Add the melted butter and toss until the mixture resembles coarse crumbs.
4. Place the haddock on a baking sheet and spoon the bread crumb mixture on top, pressing down firmly.
5. Bake the haddock in the oven for about 20 minutes or until the fish is just Cooked through and flakes off in chunks when pressed.

Per Serving
Calorie 1| Fats g| Carbs g| Protein g

Chicken Gruyere with Mushrooms

Prep time: 15 minute | Cook time: 30 minute | Serves 2

2 garlic cloves, chopped
1 chicken, skin and bone-in
3 Tablespoon ghee
8 ounces mushrooms, sliced
2 Tablespoon gruyere cheese, grated
Table salt and black pepper to the taste

1. Warm up a dish with 1 Tablespoon ghee over moderate warmth, embed chicken, season with table salt and pepper, get ready for 3 minutes on each side and organize them in a heating dish.
2. Warm up the dish again with the remainder of the ghee over moderate warmth, embed garlic, shake and plan for 1 minute.
3. Supplement mushrooms and shake well.
4. Addition table salt and pepper shake and get ready for 10 minutes.
5. Spoon these over chickens, Garnish cheddar, present in the stove at 350 degrees F and heat for 20 minutes.
6. Go stove to oven and cook everything for a couple more minutes.
7. Appropriate among plates and serve.

Per Serving
Calorie 1192| Fats 88.28g| Carbs 16.3g| Protein 83.14g

Quinoa with Peppery Oyster Mushrooms

Prep time: 15 minute | Cook time: 30 minute | Serves 4

2 1/4 cups water, divided
1 cup uncooked quinoa
3 Tablespoons olive oil
1 Tablespoon avocado oil
2 medium shallots, peeled and minced
2 cloves garlic, peeled and minced
1 cup sliced cremini mushrooms
1 cup sliced oyster mushrooms
1 cup sliced shiitake mushrooms
2 cups chopped kale
1 cup chopped Swiss chard
1 cup baby spinach leaves
2 Tablespoons lemon juice
1/2 teaspoon salt
1/8 teaspoon ground black pepper

1. Fill medium pot with 2 cups water, add quinoa, and bring to a boil. When water boils, reduce heat to low and cover; simmer covered for 12 minutes.
2. Remove from heat and keep covered an additional 5 minutes; then fluff with a fork and set aside.
3. In a large skillet, heat olive oil and avocado oil over medium heat.
4. Add shallots and garlic; cook and stir for 2 minutes.
5. Add mushrooms; cook and stir until mushrooms give up their liquid, the liquid evaporates, and they start to brown, about 8–10 minutes.
6. Add kale, Swiss chard, and remaining 1/4 cup water; cover and steam for 2 minutes.
7. Remove cover; add spinach, lemon juice, salt, and black pepper.
8. Stir, cover, and steam for another 2–4 minutes or until greens are tender and Serve.

Per Serving
Calorie 1193| Fats 65.83g| Carbs 126.67g| Protein 30.72g

Marinated Steak Skewers with Chimichurri Sauce

Prep time: 15 minute | Cook time: 30 minute | Serves 4

1 pound tri-tip steak, cut into 1" cubes
1 teaspoon salt
1/4 teaspoon ground black pepper
1 medium red bell pepper, seeded and cut into large chunks
1 medium yellow bell pepper, seeded and cut into large chunks
1 medium red onion, peeled and cut into eighths
2 Tablespoons olive oil
1/2 cup Chimichurri Sauce

1. If using bamboo skewers, soak in cool water for 25 minutes to prevent burning.
2. Season steak with salt and black pepper.
3. Thread steak and vegetables onto bamboo or metal skewers, alternating the produce. Brush with olive oil.
4. Prepare the grill on high heat.
5. Grill the steaks to desired doneness, about 2 to 3 minutes per side for medium-rare.
6. Brush with chimichurri sauce, grill for 1 more minute, then serve.

Per Serving
Calorie 443| Fats 34g| Carbs 9g| Protein 25g

Grandma's Special Spinach Artichokes Stuff

Prep time: 15 minute | Cook time: 30 minute | Serves 4

2 large artichokes	4 Tablespoons chopped fresh parsley
1/4 cup lemon juice	
2 Tablespoons avocado oil	1/2 teaspoon ground black pepper
2 cloves garlic, peeled and chopped	2 cups chopped spinach
1/2 large sweet onion, peeled and chopped	4 quarts plus 1/2 cup water, divided
1 cup almond meal	Juice and rind of 1/2 lemon
1 Tablespoon minced lemon peel	1/2 teaspoon ground coriander

1. Remove any tough or brown outside leaves from artichokes. Using a sharp knife, cut off artichoke tops, about 1/2" down.
2. Slam artichokes against a countertop to loosen leaves. Cut in half, from top to stem, and remove the thistly choke with a spoon. Trim the stem end.
3. Place in a large bowl of cold water mixed with 1/4 cup lemon juice; set aside.
4. Heat avocado oil in a large skillet over medium heat.
5. Add garlic and onion and sauté for 5 minutes, stirring.
6. Add almond meal, lemon peel, parsley, and black pepper. Cook 2 minutes.
7. Add spinach and stir until wilted, about 1 minute. Remove from heat and set aside.
8. Boil artichokes in 4 quarts water with juice and rind of 1/2 lemon, and coriander for 18 minutes.
9. Remove artichokes but reserve the cooking water.
10. Place artichokes cut side up in a baking dish with 1/2 cup water on the bottom.
11. Stuff each half with spinach mixture.
12. Preheat oven to 375°F. Drizzle stuffed artichokes with a bit of the cooking water and bake for 10 minutes until filling is browned on top and Serve.

Per Serving
Calorie 280| Fats 21g| Carbs 20g| Protein 10g

Hot Sweet Potato Vegetable Pasta

Prep time: 15 minute | Cook time: 30 minute | Serves 4

2 Tablespoons olive oil	cut into thin strips
2 large sweet potatoes, peeled and	1/2 teaspoon salt
	1/4 cup Basic Vegetable Stock

1. Heat olive oil in a large saucepan over medium-high heat.
2. Add sweet potatoes and salt; cook and stir until almost tender, about 4 minutes.
3. 2 Add stock and bring to a simmer; simmer for 2–3 minutes or until pasta is tender.
4. Serve immediately

Per Serving
Calorie 127| Fats 7g| Carbs 16g| Protein 1g

Chilly Scallion Chicken

Prep time: 15 minute | Cook time: 30 minute | Serves 3

3 Tablespoon rice vinegar	Table salt and black pepper to the taste
3 Tablespoon stevia	3 Tablespoon coconut amino
¼ mug scallions, sliced off	
½ tsp. xanthan gum	2 teaspoons white vinegar
1 pounds chicken wings	5 dried chillies, sliced off

1. Scatter chicken wings on a lined baking sheet, season with table salt and pepper, introduce within the oven at 375 degrees F and bake for 20 minutes.
2. Meanwhile, heat up a small dish over moderate heat, insert white vinegar, rice vinegar, coconut amino, stevia, xanthan gum, scallions and chillies,
3. Shake well, bring to a boil, prepare for 2 minutes and take away heat. Dip chicken wings into this sauce, organize all of them on the baking sheet again and bake for 10 minutes additional.
4. Serve them heat.

Per Serving
Calorie 611| Fats 16.24g| Carbs 6.71g| Protein 100.95g

Ground Pork and Garlic Mushrooms with Shirataki Noodles

Prep time: 15 minute | Cook time: 25 minute | Serves 4

2 Tablespoons sesame oil
1 (8-ounce) package sliced cremini mushrooms
3 cloves garlic, peeled and minced
3 Tablespoons coconut amino
1 cup Basic Vegetable

Stock
1 Tablespoon lemon juice
1/2 teaspoon ground white pepper
4 (7-ounce) packages shirataki noodles
1 pound ground pork
2 Tablespoons toasted sesame seeds

1. In a large saucepan, heat sesame oil over medium heat.
2. Add mushrooms and garlic; cook and stir until mushrooms give up their liquid and liquid evaporates, about 7 minutes.
3. Add coconut amino, stock, lemon juice, and white pepper and simmer for 8 minutes.
4. Meanwhile, cook noodles in boiling water based on package instructions. When done, drain noodles and rinse with hot water; drain again.
5. Meanwhile, heat large skillet over medium-high heat. Add pork and cook, stirring and breaking up the meat, for 6–8 minutes or until meat is cooked through. Remove pork from skillet.
6. Reduce heat to medium-high and add noodles to skillet. Cook and stir until noodles are dry.
7. Place noodles in a medium serving bowl and mix with ground pork and mushroom sauce.
8. Sprinkle with sesame seeds. Serve immediately.

Per Serving
Calorie 484| Fats 34g| Carbs 14g| Protein 34g

Homemade White pepper Tomato Pasta

Prep time: 15 minute | Cook time: 30 minute | Serves 4

2 large zucchini
14 medium Roma tomatoes, sliced
1 medium onion, peeled and chopped
2 cloves garlic, peeled and sliced
2 Tablespoons olive oil
1/2 teaspoon salt
1/8 teaspoon ground

white pepper
1 Tablespoon maple syrup
1 Tablespoon grass-fed butter
1 teaspoon dried oregano
1/2 teaspoon dried basil
1/2 teaspoon dried thyme

1. Cut zucchini into noodle-shaped strips using a sharp knife or a spiral cutter, avoiding the seed center. Set aside.
2. Preheat oven to 325°F. Place tomatoes on a large rimmed baking sheet. Sprinkle with onion, garlic, olive oil, salt, and white pepper. Drizzle with maple syrup.
3. Roast tomatoes for 11/2 hours or until they start to break down and look brown around the edges.
4. In a large saucepan, heat butter.
5. Sauté zucchini noodles for 2–3 minutes or until tender.
6. Add tomatoes and all scrapings from the baking sheet used to roast the tomatoes along with oregano, basil, and thyme; cook and stir for 1 minute longer. Serve immediately.

Per Serving
Calorie 218| Fats 12g| Carbs 28g| Protein 6g

Grandma's spaghetti Chicken Recipe

Prep time: 15 minute | Cook time: 30 minute | Serves 6

¼ mug parmesan, grated
½ tsp. garlic grinding grains
1 and ½ teaspoons parsley, dried
½ tsp. basil, dried
4 Tablespoon avocado oil
1 and ½ pounds chicken breast, skinless and boneless and cubed
Table salt and black pepper to the taste
1 egg
1 mug almond flour
4 mugs spaghetti squash, already prepared
6 ounces mozzarella, shredded
1 and ½ mugs marinara sauce
Fresh basil, sliced off for serving

1. In a pot, consolidate almond flour with pram, table salt, pepper, garlic granulating grains and 1 tsp. parsley and shake.
2. In another pot, whisk the egg with a spot of table salt and pepper and dunk chicken in egg and afterward in almond flour consolidate.
3. Warm up a dish with 3 Tablespoon oil over moderate gigantic warmth, embed chicken, get ready until they are brilliant on the two sides and move to paper towels.
4. In a pot, consolidate spaghetti squash with table salt, pepper, dried basil, 1 Tablespoon oil and the remainder of the parsley and shake.
5. Disperse this into a heatproof dish, embed chicken pieces and afterward the marinara sauce.
6. Top with destroyed mozzarella, present in the broiler at 375 degrees F and prepare for 30 minutes.
7. Embellishment new basil toward the end, leave dish aside to chill off a piece, conveys among plates and serves.

Per Serving
Calorie 1673| Fats 108.32g| Carbs 12.22g| Protein 158.84g

Curried Shrimp and Cauliflower with Cilantro

Prep time: 15 minute | Cook time: 30 minute | Serves 4

3/4 cup Basic Vegetable Stock (see recipe in Chapter 6)
1 cup canned full-fat coconut milk
11/2 cups chopped green beans
1 small head cauliflower, chopped
2 medium carrots, peeled and diced
2 teaspoons minced fresh ginger
3 cloves garlic, peeled
and minced
2 teaspoons curry powder
1/2 teaspoon turmeric
1 Tablespoon maple syrup
1/4 teaspoon salt
1/4 teaspoon nutmeg
1 pound large shrimp, peeled and deveined, tails on
2 Tablespoons chopped fresh cilantro

1. Whisk together vegetable stock and coconut milk in a large saucepan.
2. Add remaining ingredients except for shrimp and cilantro, stirring well to combine.
3. Bring to a slow simmer over low heat, cover, and cook for 5–6 minutes, stirring occasionally.
4. Add shrimp and cook until shrimp are bright pink and cooked through, 5–6 more minutes.
5. Top with cilantro and serve hot.

Per Serving
Calorie 181| Fats 10g| Carbs 15g| Protein 9g

CHAPTER 6: SMOOTHIES AND DRINKS

Zero Fat Romaine Lettuce Smoothie

Prep time: 15 minutes | Cook time: 0 minutes | Serves 2

1 cup chopped romaine lettuce
2 medium cucumbers,
peeled and quartered
1/4 cup chopped mint
1 cup water, divided

1. Place romaine, cucumbers, mint, and 1/2 cup water in a blender and combine thoroughly.
2. Add remaining water while blending until desired texture is achieved.

Per Serving

Calorie 40| Fat 0g| Carbs 9g| Protein 2g

Classic Almond Banana Date Shake

Prep time: 15 minutes | Cook time: 0 minutes | Serves 2

2 Tablespoon almond butter
1 tablespoon egg white grinding grains
1 tablespoon unsweetened cocoa grinding grains (optional)
½ Teaspoon. fresh lemon juice
⅓ Mug sliced off, pitted Medjool dates
1 mug unsweetened almond or coconut milk (with vanilla if desired)
1 ripe banana, frozen and sliced
⅛ Teaspoon ground nutmeg

1. In a small pot combine date and ½ mug water.
2. Microwave on immense for 30 seconds or until dates are softened; drain off water.
3. In a blender combine the dates, almond milk, banana slices, almond butter, egg white grinding grains, cocoa grinding grains (if using), lemon juice, and nutmeg.
4. Wrap up and blend until smooth.

Per Serving

Calorie 247| Fat 23.9g| Carbs 9.52g| Protein3.04g

Sweet and Creamy Banana Apricot Smoothie

Prep time: 15 minutes | Cook time: 0 minutes | Serves 2

3 medium apricots, pitted
1 medium banana, peeled
1/2 cup water
1/2 cup canned full-fat coconut milk
4–6 ice cubes

1. Combine all ingredients in a blender and blend until smooth and frosty

Per Serving

Calorie 320| Fat 17g| Carbs 38g| Protein 4g

Strawberry- Pomegranate Smoothie

Prep time: 10 minutes | Cook time: 30 minutes | Serves 2

1¼ mugs unsweetened coconut milk or almond milk
¼ mug unsweetened pomegranate juice
¼ mug unable salted almond butter
1 moderate red beet, peeled and quartered
(about 4 ounces)
2½ mugs hulled fresh strawberries
1½ mugs frozen unsweetened mango chunks
2 teaspoons egg white grinding grains

1. In a moderate sauce dish prepare beet, Wrap upped, in a small amount of boiling water for 30 minutes or until very tender.
2. Drain beet; run cold water over beet to cool quickly and drain well.
3. In a blender combine beet, strawberries, mango chunks, coconut milk, pomegranate juice, and almond butter.
4. Wrap up and blend until smooth, stopping to scrape sides of blender as needed. Insert egg white grinding grains.
5. Wrap up and blend just until combined. Shift frozen mango pieces to an airtight container; freeze for up to 3 months.

Per Serving

Calorie 50| Fat 0.25g| Carbs 10.22g| Protein 2.62g

Vanilla flavoured Oatmeal Smoothie

Prep time: 15 minutes | Cook time: 0 minutes | Serves 2

2 tablespoons rolled oats	2 medium apples, cored and peeled
1 cup chopped watercress	2 cups unsweetened vanilla almond milk, divided
2 medium peaches, pitted	

1. Place oats, watercress, peaches, apples, and 1 cup almond milk in a blender and blend until thoroughly combined.
2. Add remaining almond milk while blending until desired texture is achieved.

Per Serving

Calorie 198| Fat 4g| Carbs 43g| Protein 4g

Spinach Zucchini Green Smoothie

Prep time: 15 minutes | Cook time: 0 minutes | Serves 2

1 cup spinach	peeled and chopped
1 medium zucchini, chopped	2 medium apples, cored and peeled
3 medium carrots,	2 cups water, divided

1. Place spinach, zucchini, carrots, apples, and 1 cup water in a blender and blend until thoroughly combined.
2. Add remaining water while blending until desired texture is achieved.

Per Serving

Calorie 163| Fat 1g| Carbs 40g| Protein 4g

Clear Your Mind Lettuce Smoothie

Prep time: 15 minutes | Cook time: 0 minutes | Serves 2

1 cup chopped romaine lettuce	1 medium cucumber, chopped
2 medium tomatoes	1/2 cup chopped green onions
1 medium zucchini, chopped	2 cloves garlic, peeled
2 medium stalks celery, chopped	2 cups water, divided

1. Place romaine, tomatoes, zucchini, celery, cucumber, green onions, garlic, and 1 cup water in a blender and blend until thoroughly combined.
2. Add remaining 1 cup water, if needed, while blending until desired texture is achieved.

Per Serving

Calorie 86| Fat 1g| Carbs 17g| Protein 5g

Homemade zucchini Carrot Smoothie

Prep time: 15 minutes | Cook time: 0 minutes | Serves 2

1 cup chopped romaine lettuce	chopped
1 cup chopped broccoli	2 medium carrots, peeled and chopped
1 medium zucchini,	2 cups water, divided

1. Place romaine, broccoli, zucchini, carrots, and 1 cup water in a blender and blend until thoroughly combined.
2. Add remaining water while blending until desired texture is achieved.

Per Serving

Calorie 71| Fat 1g| Carbs 15g| Protein 4g

Lemony Grapefruit Watercress Smoothie

Prep time: 15 minutes | Cook time: 0 minutes | Serves 2

1 cup chopped watercress	1 (1/2") piece gingerroot, peeled
1 large grapefruit, peeled	1/2 medium lemon, peeled
2 medium oranges, peeled	1 cup water, divided

1. Place watercress, grapefruit, oranges, gingerroot, lemon, and 1/2 cup water in a blender and blend until thoroughly combined.
2. Add remaining water while blending until desired texture is achieved.

Per Serving

Calorie 136| Fat 0g| Carbs 35g| Protein 3g

Healthy Watercress Orange Smoothie

Prep time: 15 minutes | Cook time: 0 minutes | Serves 2

2 Cup chopped watercress
2 medium oranges, peeled
1 cup strawberries

1 cup blueberries
1 cup water
1 cup canned full-fat coconut milk, divided

1. Place watercress, oranges, strawberries, blueberries, water and 1/2 cup coconut milk in a blender and blend until thoroughly combined.
2. Add remaining coconut milk while blending until desired texture is achieved.

Per Serving
Calorie 310| Fat 15g| Carbs 35g| Protein 4g

Homemade Lettuce Carrot Smoothie

Prep time: 15 minutes | Cook time: 0 minutes | Serves 2

2 cups chopped romaine lettuce
3 medium carrots, peeled and chopped

1 medium apple, peeled and cored
1 cup water

1. Combine all ingredients except water in a blender.
2. Add water slowly while blending until desired texture is achieved.

Per Serving
Calorie 93| Fat 1g| Carbs 23g| Protein 2g

Glowing Lettuce Banana Smoothie

Prep time: 15 minutes | Cook time: 0 minutes | Serves 3

4 cups chopped romaine lettuce
4 medium pears, cored
1 medium banana,

peeled
6 tablespoons lemon juice
2 cups water, divided

1. Place romaine, pears, banana, lemon juice, and 1 cup water in a blender and blend until thoroughly combined.

2. Add remaining water while blending until desired texture is achieved.

Per Serving
Calorie 183| Fat 1g| Carbs 48g| Protein 2g

Chilled Three Pears - Banana Smoothie

Prep time: 15 minutes | Cook time: 0 minutes | Serves 2

3 medium pears, peeled, cored, and sliced
1 banana, peeled

1 cup unsweetened vanilla almond milk
1 teaspoon cinnamon
2 cups ice, divided

1. Preheat oven to 375°F.
2. Layer pears in a shallow baking dish.
3. Add enough water to cover the bottom of the baking dish, and bake for 20 minutes or until pears are fork tender.
4. Combine pears, banana, almond milk, and cinnamon in a blender with 1/2 cup ice and blend until thoroughly combined.
5. Add remaining ice gradually while blending until desired consistency is reached.

Per Serving
Calorie 215| Fat 2g| Carbs 53g| Protein 2g

Lettuce & Double Berry Smoothie

Prep time: 15 minutes | Cook time: 0 minutes | Serves 2

1 cup chopped romaine lettuce
2 medium bananas, peeled
1 pint strawberries

1 pint blueberries
2 cups unsweetened vanilla almond milk, divided

1. Place romaine, bananas, berries, and 1 cup almond milk in a blender and blend until thoroughly combined.
2. Add remaining almond milk while blending until desired texture is achieved.

Per Serving
Calorie 211| Fat 4g| Carbs 46g| Protein 4g

Vanilla Almond Apple Smoothie

Prep time: 15 minutes | Cook time: 0 minutes | Serves 2

2 cups spinach	cored and peeled
1 medium banana, peeled	2 cups unsweetened vanilla almond milk, divided
2 medium apples,	

1. Place spinach, banana, apples, and 1 cup almond milk in a blender and blend until thoroughly combined.
2. Add remaining almond milk while blending until desired texture is achieved.

Per Serving

Calorie 183| Fat 3g| Carbs 39g| Protein 3g

Vanilla flavoured Banana Smoothie

Prep time: 15 minutes | Cook time: 0 minutes | Serves 2

1 cup chopped romaine lettuce	powder
2 medium bananas, peeled	1/2 teaspoon vanilla bean pulp
1 tablespoon cocoa	2 cups oat milk, divided

1. Place romaine, bananas, cocoa powder, vanilla bean pulp, and 1 cup oat milk in a blender and blend until thoroughly combined.
2. Add remaining oat milk while blending until desired texture is achieved.

Per Serving

Calorie 230| Fat 3g| Carbs 49g| Protein 7g

Feel Clean Banana- Dandelion Detox Smoothie

Prep time: 15 minutes | Cook time: 0 minutes | Serves 2

1/2 cup chopped dandelion greens	1 medium banana, peeled
1/2 cup arugula	1 cup water
2 cups chopped pineapple	1 cup canned full-fat coconut milk, divided

1. Place dandelion greens, arugula, and pineapple, banana, water and 1/2 cup coconut milk in a blender and blend until thoroughly combined.
2. Add remaining coconut milk while blending until desired texture is achieved.

Per Serving

Calorie 315| Fat 17g| Carbs38g| Protein 3g

Grapefruit Watercress Super Smoothie

Prep time: 15 minutes | Cook time: 0 minutes | Serves 2

1 cup chopped watercress	peeled
1 large grapefruit, peeled	1 medium banana, peeled
2 medium oranges,	1 cup water, divided

1. Place watercress, grapefruit, oranges, banana, and 1/2 cup water in a blender and blend until thoroughly combined.
2. Add remaining water while blending until desired texture is achieved.

Per Serving

Calorie 162| Fat 1g| Carbs 41g| Protein 3g

Six Ingredients- Feel Fresh Smoothie

Prep time: 15 minutes | Cook time: 0 minutes | Serves 2

1 cup chopped iceberg lettuce	cherries
2 medium pears, cored	1/2 teaspoon vanilla bean pulp
1 medium banana, peeled	2 cups unsweetened vanilla almond milk, divided
1/2 cup pitted	

1. Place lettuce, pears, banana, cherries, vanilla bean pulp, and 1 cup almond milk in a blender and blend until thoroughly combined.
2. Add remaining almond milk while blending until desired texture is achieved.

Per Serving

Calorie 216| Fat 3g| Carbs 48g| Protein 3g

Four Ingredients Ginger Lemon Water

Prep time: 15 minutes | Cook time: 15 minutes | Serves 6

5 cups water
3/4 cup lemon juice
3/4 cup maple syrup

½ piece gingerroot, peeled and sliced

1. Combine all ingredients in a 2-quart or smaller slow cooker.
2. Cover and cook on high for 15 minutes (if mixture begins to boil, turn heat to low).
3. Chill and serve over ice.
4. Remove gingerroot before serving.

Per Serving
Calorie 109| Fat 0g| Carbs 29g| Protein 0g

Detoxifying Spicy Black Tea

Prep time: 15 minutes | Cook time: 30 minutes | Serves 22

5 cups water
6 slices fresh ginger
1 teaspoon whole cloves
2 (3") cinnamon sticks
11/2 teaspoons freshly ground

nutmeg
1/2 teaspoon ground cardamom
1 cup maple syrup
12 bags black tea
6 cups unsweetened vanilla almond milk

1. Pour water into a 4-quart slow cooker.
2. Put ginger and cloves in a muslin spice bag or a piece of cheese cloth secured with a piece of kitchen twine
3. Add to the cooker along with cinnamon sticks, nutmeg, and cardamom.
4. Cover and cook on low for 15 minutes.
5. Stir in maple syrup until it's dissolved into the water.
6. Add tea bags and almond milk; cover and cook on low for 15 minutes.
7. Remove and discard the spices in the muslin bag or cheesecloth, the cinnamon sticks, and the tea bags.
8. Ladle into teacups or mugs to serve.

Per Serving
Calorie 88| Fat 1g| Carbs 19g| Protein 1g

Natural Vanilla Avocado Smoothie

Prep time: 15 minutes | Cook time: 0 minutes | Serves 2

1 large ripe avocado, pitted and peeled
1 cup unsweetened vanilla almond milk

1/2 cup water
2 tablespoons maple syrup
3–4 ice cubes

1. Combine all ingredients in a blender and blend until smooth.
2. Serve chilled.

Per Serving
Calorie 365| Fat 24g| Carbs 39g| Protein 4g

Spinach Tomato Blast Smoothie

Prep time: 15 minutes | Cook time: 0 minutes | Serves 2

1 cup spinach
1 medium tomato
1 medium stalk celery, chopped

2 tablespoons cilantro
1 clove garlic, peeled
2 cups water, divided

1. Place spinach, tomato, celery, cilantro, garlic, and 1 cup water in a blender and blend until thoroughly combined.
2. Add remaining 1 cup water while blending until desired texture is achieved.

Per Serving
Calorie 51| Fat 1g| Carbs 10g| Protein 3g

Coconut Milk Shake with Cocoa Nibs

Prep time: 15 minutes | Cook time: 0 minutes | Serves 2

1/3 cup canned full-fat coconut milk
2/3 cup water
1/4 cup cacao nibs
1 tablespoon honey

1/2 teaspoon cinnamon
1/4 teaspoon nutmeg
4–6 ice cubes

1. Combine all ingredients in a blender and purée until smooth.

Per Serving
Calorie 365| Fat 25g| Carbs 27g| Protein 5g

Avocado Nutmeg Oat Milk Smoothie

Prep time: 15 minutes | Cook time: 0 minutes | Serves 2

1 cup frozen blueberries
1/2 medium avocado, peeled and pitted
1 cup oat milk

1 cup spinach
1/8 teaspoon ground nutmeg
4–6 ice cubes

1. Combine all ingredients in a blender and purée until smooth.

Per Serving

Calorie 367| Fat 14g| Carbs 59g| Protein 8g

Sweet Roma Tomato Double Berry Smoothie

Prep time: 10 minutes | Cook time: 0 minutes | Serves 3

1 cup sliced strawberries
1 cup raspberries
1 medium Roma tomato, seeded and chopped

1 cup unsweetened rice milk
1 tablespoon maple syrup
1/2 teaspoon vanilla
3 ice cubes

1. Combine all ingredients in a blender and blend until smooth.
2. Pour immediately into glasses and serve.

Per Serving

Calorie 82| Fat 2g| Carbs 18g| Protein 2g

Apple Banana Protein Smoothie

Prep time: 10 minutes | Cook time: 0 minutes | Serves 2

2 cups spinach
1 medium banana, peeled
2 medium apples,

cored and peeled
2 cups unsweetened vanilla almond milk, divided

1. Place spinach, banana, apples, and 1 cup almond milk in a blender and blend until thoroughly combined.
2. Add remaining almond milk while blending until desired texture is achieved.

Per Serving

Calorie 183| Fat 3g| Carbs 39g| Protein 3g

Four Ingredient Healthy Orange water

Prep time: 15 minutes | Cook time: 15 minutes | Serves 6

5 cups water
Juice from 5 large oranges

1/2 cup maple syrup
½ piece gingerroot, peeled and sliced

1. Combine all ingredients in a 2-quart slow cooker.
2. Cover and cook on high for 15 minutes (if mixture begins to boil, turn heat to low).
3. Allow cooling and serving chilled. (Remove gingerroot before serving)

Per Serving

Calorie 100| Fat 0g| Carbs 25g| Protein 0g

Herbal Cinnamon Tea

Prep time: 15 minutes | Cook time: 5 minutes | Serves 6

4 bags herbal tea
1 teaspoon ground nutmeg
1/2 teaspoon ground

cinnamon
1/4 teaspoon ground cloves
5 cups boiling water

1. In a ceramic teapot, combine tea bags and spices.
2. Pour boiling water into teapot.
3. Steep for 5 minutes, then remove tea bags

Per Serving

Calorie 6| Fat 0g| Carbs 0g| Protein0g

Tasty Raspberry Mango Smoothie

Prep time: 10 minutes | Cook time: 0 minutes | Serves 2

1 cup chopped watercress
1 medium mango, pitted and peeled

1 cup raspberries
11/2 cups oat milk, divided

1. Place watercress, mango, raspberries, and 3/4 cup oat milk in a blender and blend until thoroughly combined.
2. Add remaining oat milk while blending until desired texture is achieved.

Per Serving

Calorie 232| Fat 3g| Carbs 50g| Protein 6g

Spinach Zucchini Smoothie

Prep time: 10 minutes | Cook time: 0 minutes | Serves 2

1 cup spinach
1 medium zucchini, chopped
3 medium carrots,

peeled and chopped
2 medium apples, cored and peeled
2 cups water, divided

1. Place spinach, zucchini, carrots, apples, and 1 cup water in a blender and blend until thoroughly combined.
2. Add remaining water while blending until desired texture is achieved.

Per Serving

Calorie 163| Fat 1g| Carbs 40g| Protein 4g

Broccoli Zucchini Smoothie

Prep time: 10 minutes | Cook time: 0 minutes | Serves 2

1 cup chopped romaine lettuce
1 cup chopped broccoli
1 medium zucchini,

chopped
2 medium carrots, peeled and chopped
2 cups water, divided

1. Place romaine, broccoli, zucchini, carrots, and 1 cup water in a blender and blend until thoroughly combined.
2. Add remaining water while blending until desired texture is achieved.

Per Serving

Calorie 71| Fat 1g| Carbs 15g| Protein 4g

Cranberry Cocktail Recipe

Prep time: 10 minutes | Cook time: 0 minutes | Serves 2

¼ cup cranberry juice cocktail
2/3 cup silken tofu, firm
½ cup raspberries,

frozen, unsweetened
½ cup blueberries, frozen, unsweetened
1 teaspoon vanilla extract

1. Pour juice into a blender. Add rest of ingredients. Blend until very smooth.
2. Serve immediately and enjoy!

Per Serving

Calorie 440| Fat 3.8g| Carbs 95.24g| Protein 8.04g

Banana Yogurt -Oat bran Smoothie

Prep time: 10 minutes | Cook time: 0 minutes | Serves 2

½ banana, peeled and cut into chunks
½ cup plain yogurt
½ cup applesauce, unsweetened

¼ cup almond or rice milk
1 tablespoon honey
2 tablespoons oat or wheat bran

1. Place banana, yogurt, applesauce, milk and honey in blender.
2. Blend until smooth.
3. Add oat bran and blend until thickened.

Per Serving

Calorie 236| Fat 5.62g| Carbs 44.4g| Protein 7.67g

Healthy Spicy Cranberry- Dates Juice

Prep time: 10 minutes | Cook time: 0 minutes | Serves 2

1 cup organic cranberries
4 cups of filtered water, divided
4 dates or 2 Tablespoon date paste or 2 Tablespoon maple syrup
2 red organic apples,

sliced
Juice of 2 organic lemons
1 Teaspoon Cardamom (optional)
1 sprig fresh organic mint or peppermint (optional)

1. In a medium size pot combines the cranberries and 3 cups of water and brings to a boil.
2. Turn the heat off and let cool. In a food processor blend the dates or date paste with lemon juice and remaining one cup of water.
3. Transfer to a large glass container or jar and add sliced apples, and all the cranberries and water.
4. Stir and add cardamom and mint leaves if desired.

Per Serving

Calorie 622| Fat 1.51g| Carbs 155.45g| Protein 1.73g

Vanilla Whey Protein Drink

Prep time: 10 minutes | Cook time: 0 minutes | Serves 2

3/4 cup pineapple sherbet or sorbet	protein powder
1 scoop vanilla whey	1/2 cup water
	2 ice cubes, optional

1. In a blender, add pineapple sherbet, whey protein powder and water (ice cubes optional).
2. Immediately blend for 30 to 45 seconds.

Per Serving

Calorie 215| Fat 0.48g| Carbs 37.67g| Protein 17.47g

Easy Tasty Banana Date Smoothie

Prep time: 15 minutes | Cook time: 0 minutes | Serves 2

3 large pitted dates	1 medium banana, peeled
Water for soaking	6 ice cubes
3/4 cup unsweetened vanilla almond milk	1/4 teaspoon vanilla

1. In a small bowl, cover dates with water and soak for at least 10 minutes.
2. Discard soaking water and add dates and all other ingredients to a lender.
3. Process about 1 minute on medium speed until smooth.

Per Serving

Calorie 177| Fat 2g| Carbs 40g| Protein 3g

Tasty Banana Mango Fruit Drink

Prep time: 15 minutes | Cook time: 0 minutes | Serves 2

1 cup chopped mango	1 cup unsweetened vanilla almond milk
1 large banana, peeled	2 cups ice, divided

1. Combine mango, banana, and almond milk in a blender with 1/2 cup ice and blend until thoroughly combined.
2. Add remaining ice gradually while blending until desired consistency is reached.

Per Serving

Calorie 132| Fat 2g| Carbs 30g| Protein 2g

Healthy Frozen Coconut Smoothie

Prep time: 15 minutes | Cook time: 0 minutes | Serves 2

11/2 cups mashed and softened coconut meat	mango
	1 medium clementine, peeled
1 cup chopped pineapple	2 cups unsweetened almond milk
1/2 cup chopped	2 cups ice, divided

1. Combine coconut, pineapple, mango, clementine, and almond milk in a blender with 1/2 cup ice, and blend until thoroughly combined.
2. Add remaining ice gradually while blending until desired consistency is reached.

Per Serving

Calorie 416| Fat 30g| Carbs 38g| Protein 5g

Chilled and Creamy Berry Dessert

Prep time: 15 minutes | Cook time: 10 minutes | Serves 2

1 cup vanilla rice milk, at room temperature	cinnamon
1/2 cup plain cream cheese, at room temperature	1 cup crumbled Meringue Cookies
	2 cups fresh blueberries
1 tablespoon granulated sugar	1 cup sliced fresh strawberries
1/2 teaspoon ground	

1. In a small bowl, whisk together the milk, cream cheese, sugar, and cinnamon until smooth.
2. Into 4 (6-ounce) glasses, spoon 1/4 cup of crumbled cookie in the bottom of each.
3. Spoon 1/4 cup of the cream cheese mixture on top of the cookies.
4. Top the cream cheese with 1/4 cup of the berries.
5. Repeat in each cup with the cookies, cream cheese mixture, and berries.
6. Chill in the refrigerator for 1 hour and serve.

Per Serving

Calorie 1624| Fat 59.25g| Carbs 258.99g| Protein 29.03g

Very Cherry Banana Smoothie

Prep time: 15 minutes | Cook time: 0 minutes | Serves 2

2 cups pitted cherries
1 medium banana, peeled
1 cup kale
Pulp of 1 vanilla bean
1 cup unsweetened vanilla almond milk
1 teaspoon vanilla extract
1 cup ice, divided

1. Combine cherries, banana, kale, vanilla bean pulp, almond milk, and vanilla extract in the blender with 1/2 cup ice and blend until thoroughly combined.
2. Add remaining ice gradually while blending until desired consistency is reached.

Per Serving

Calorie 170| Fat 2g| Carbs 38g| Protein 3g

Beets and Carrot Smoothie

Prep time: 15 minutes | Cook time: 0 minutes | Serves 2

1 cup chopped beet greens
2 medium beets, peeled and chopped
2 medium carrots,
peeled and chopped
1 medium cucumber, peeled and chopped
2 cups water, divided

1. Place beet greens, beets, carrots, cucumber, and 1 cup water in a blender and blend until thoroughly combined.
2. Add remaining 1 cup water while blending until desired texture is achieved.

Per Serving

Calorie 87| Fat 1g| Carbs 20g| Protein 3g

Homemade Vanilla Hot Cereal

Prep time: 15 minutes | Cook time: 10 minutes | Serves 2

2¼ cups water
1¼ cups vanilla rice milk
6 tablespoons uncooked bulgur
2 tablespoons uncooked whole
buckwheat
1 cup peeled, sliced apple
6 tablespoons plain uncooked couscous
½ teaspoon ground cinnamon

1. In a medium saucepan over medium-high heat, heat the water and milk.
2. Bring to a boil, and add the bulgur, buckwheat, and apple.
3. Reduce the heat to low and simmer, stirring occasionally, for 20 to 25 minutes or until the bulgur is tender.
4. Remove the saucepan from the heat and stir in the couscous and cinnamon.
5. Let the saucepan stand, covered, for 10 minutes, and then fluff the cereal with a fork before serving.

Per Serving

Calorie 476| Fat 1.89g| Carbs 105.61g| Protein 12.15g

Grandma's Tasty Corn Pudding

Prep time: 15 minutes | Cook time: 10 minutes | Serves 2

Unsalted butter, for greasing the baking dish
2 tablespoons all-purpose flour
½ teaspoon Ener-G baking soda substitute
3 eggs
¾ cup unsweetened rice milk, at room
temperature
3 tablespoons unsalted butter, melted
2 tablespoons light sour cream
2 tablespoons granulated sugar
2 cups frozen corn kernels, thawed

1. Preheat the oven to 350°F.
2. Lightly grease an 8-by-8-inch baking dish with butter; set aside.
3. In a small bowl, stir together the flour and baking soda substitute; set aside.
4. In a medium bowl, whisk together the eggs, rice milk, butter, sour cream, and sugar.
5. Stir the flour mixture into the egg mixture until smooth.
6. Add the corn to the batter and stir until very well mixed.
7. Spoon the batter into the baking dish and bake for about 40 minutes or until the pudding is set.
8. Let the pudding cool for about 15 minutes and serve warm.

Per Serving

Calorie 1358| Fat 65.11g| Carbs 142.51g| Protein 48.52g

Vegan Vanilla Cashew Smoothie

Prep time: 15 minutes | Cook time: 0 minutes | Serves 2

1 cup raw cashews	water for milk
Water for soaking	1/2 teaspoon salt
Additional 4 cups	1/2 teaspoon vanilla

1. In a large bowl, cover nuts with plenty of water and allow soaking for at least 1 hour or overnight. Drain.
2. Blend soaked nuts with 4 cups water in a food processor. Purée on high until smooth.
3. Strain through cheesecloth or a sieve. Stir in salt and vanilla.

Per Serving

Calorie 143| Fat 11g| Carbs 8g| Protein 5g

Healthy Peach Coconut Smoothie

Prep time: 10 minutes | Cook time: 0 minutes | Serves 2

1 large orange, peeled	peeled
1 medium peach, pitted	1 Watercress
1 medium banana,	1 cup canned full-fat coconut milk, divided

1. Place watercress, orange, peach, banana, and 1/2 cup coconut milk in a blender and blend until thoroughly combined.
2. Add remaining coconut milk while blending until desired texture is achieved.

Per Serving

Calorie 300| Fat 15g| Carbs 33g| Protein 4g

Classic Bread Pudding

Prep time: 15 minutes | Cook time: 30 minutes | Serves 2

Unsalted butter, for greasing the baking dish	1 tablespoon corn-starch
1½ cups unsweetened rice milk	1 vanilla bean, split
3 eggs	10 thick pieces white bread, cut into 1-inch chunks
½ cup granulated sugar	2 cups chopped fresh rhubarb

1. Preheat the oven to 350°F.
2. Lightly grease an 8-by-8-inch baking dish with butter; set aside.
3. In a large bowl, whisk together the rice milk, eggs, sugar, and corn starch.
4. Scrape the vanilla seeds into the milk mixture and whisk to blend.
5. Add the bread to the egg mixture and stir to completely coat the bread.
6. Add the chopped rhubarb and stir to combine.
7. Let the bread and egg mixture soak for 5 minutes.
8. Spoon the mixture into the prepared baking dish, cover with aluminum foil, and bake for 20 minutes.
9. Uncover the bread pudding and bake for an additional 10 minutes or until the pudding is golden brown and set.
10. Serve warm.

Per Serving

Calorie 1605| Fat 35.89g| Carbs 285.77g| Protein 45.03g

Apple Tea for Weight loss

Prep time: 15 minutes | Cook time: 5 minutes | Serves 2

1 cup unsweetened rice milk	1 apple, peeled, cored, and chopped
1 chai tea bag	2 cups ice

1. In a medium saucepan, heat the rice milk over low heat for about 5 minutes or until steaming.
2. Remove the milk from the heat and add the tea bag to steep.
3. Let the milk cool in the refrigerator with the tea bag for about 20 minutes and then remove tea bag, squeezing gently to release the entire flavor.
4. Place the milk, apple, and ice in a blender and blend until smooth.
5. Pour into 2 glasses and serve.

Per Serving

Calorie 243| Fat 8.29g| Carbs g| Protein 8.16g

Coconut Milk Pineapple Smoothie

Prep time: 10 minutes | Cook time: 0 minutes | Serves 2

1/2 cup chopped dandelion greens
1/2 cup arugula
2 cups chopped pineapple

1 medium banana, peeled
1 cup water
1 cup canned full-fat coconut milk, divided

1. Place dandelion greens, arugula, and pineapple, banana, water and 1/2 cup coconut milk in a blender and blend until thoroughly combined.
2. Add remaining coconut milk while blending until desired texture is achieved.

Per Serving
Calorie 315| Fat 17g| Carbs 38g| Protein 3g

Fresh Green Smoothie

Prep time: 10 minutes | Cook time: 0 minutes | Serves 1

1 cup chopped romaine lettuce
2 medium cucumbers,

peeled and quartered
1/4 cup chopped mint
1 cup water, divided

1. Place romaine, cucumbers, mint, and 1/2 cup water in a blender and combine thoroughly.
2. Add remaining water while blending until desired texture is achieved.

Per Serving
Calorie 40| Fat 0g| Carbs 9g| Protein 2g

Chocolate Oatmeal Banana Smoothie

Prep time: 10 minutes | Cook time: 0 minutes | Serves 2

1 cup chopped romaine lettuce
2 medium bananas, peeled
1 tablespoon cocoa

powder
1/2 teaspoon vanilla bean pulp
2 cups oat milk, divided

1. Place romaine, bananas, cocoa powder, vanilla bean pulp, and 1 cup oat milk in a blender and blend until thoroughly combined.

2. Add remaining oat milk while blending until desired texture is achieved.

Per Serving
Calorie 230| Fat 3g| Carbs 49g| Protein 7g

Almond Milk Cherry Smoothie

Prep time: 10 minutes | Cook time: 0 minutes | Serves 2

1 cup chopped iceberg lettuce
2 medium pears, cored
1 medium banana, peeled
1/2 cup pitted

cherries
1/2 teaspoon vanilla bean pulp
2 cups unsweetened vanilla almond milk, divided

1. Place lettuce, pears, banana, cherries, vanilla bean pulp, and 1 cup almond milk in a blender and blend until thoroughly combined.
2. Add remaining almond milk while blending until desired texture is achieved.

Per Serving
Calorie 216| Fat 3g| Carbs 48g| Protein 3g

Homemade Oats Apple Smoothie

Prep time: 10 minutes | Cook time: 0 minutes | Serves 2

2 tablespoons rolled oats
1 cup chopped watercress
2 medium peaches, pitted

2 medium apples, cored and peeled
cups unsweetened vanilla almond milk, divided

1. Place oats, watercress, peaches, apples, and 1 cup almond milk in a blender and blend until thoroughly combined.
2. Add remaining almond milk while blending until desired texture is achieved.

Per Serving
Calorie 198| Fat 4g| Carbs 43g| Protein 4g

Blueberry Pineapple Smoothie

Prep time: 15 minutes | Cook time: 0 minutes | Serves 2

1 cup frozen blueberries
½ cup pineapple chunks
½ cup English cucumber
½ apples
½ cup water

1. Put the blueberries, pineapple, cucumber, apple, and water in a blender and
2. Blend until thick and smooth.
3. Pour into 2 glasses and serve.

Per Serving

Calorie 239| Fat 1.36g| Carbs 59.91g| Protein 1.73g

Watermelon Raspberry Smoothie

Prep time: 15 minutes | Cook time: 0 minutes | Serves 2

½ cup boiled, cooled, and shredded red cabbage
1 cup diced watermelon
½ cup fresh raspberries
1 cup ice

1. Put the cabbage in a blender and pulse for 2 minutes or until it is finely chopped.
2. Add the watermelon and raspberries and pulse for about 1 minute or until very well combined.
3. Add the ice and blend until the smoothie is very thick and smooth.
4. Pour into 2 glasses and serve.

Per Serving

Calorie 176| Fat 0.46g| Carbs 44.81g| Protein 2.64g

Feel Fresh Lemony Watercress Smoothie

Prep time: 15 minutes | Cook time: 0 minutes | Serves 2

1 cup chopped watercress
1 cup chopped asparagus
1 small lemon, peeled
1 large orange, peeled
1 cup water, divided

1. Place watercress, asparagus, lemon, orange, and 1/2 cup water in a blender and blend until thoroughly combined.
2. Add remaining water while blending until desired texture is achieved.

Per Serving

Calorie 65| Fat 0g| Carbs 16g| Protein 3g

Apple & Spinach Detox Smoothie

Prep time: 15 minutes | Cook time: 0 minutes | Serves 2

1 cup spinach
2 medium green apples, peeled and cored
1/2 medium banana, peeled
1 cup water, divided

1. Place spinach, apples, banana, and 1/2 cup water in a blender and blend until thoroughly combined.
2. Continue adding remaining water while blending until desired texture is achieved

Per Serving

Calorie 241| Fat 1g| Carbs 63g| Protein 2g

Simple Raw Tomato Juice

Prep time: 15 minutes | Cook time: 20 minutes | Serves 4

10 large tomatoes, seeded and sliced
1 teaspoon lemon juice
1/4 teaspoon ground black pepper
1 tablespoon maple syrup

1. Place tomatoes in a 2-quart slow cooker and cook on low for 20 minutes.
2. Press cooked tomatoes through a sieve.
3. Add remaining ingredients and chill

Per Serving

Calorie 95| Fat 1g| Carbs 21g| Protein 4g

Watercress Peachy Banana Smoothie

Prep time: 15 minutes | Cook time: 0 minutes | Serves 2

1 cup chopped watercress
1 large orange, peeled
1 medium peach,
pitted
1 medium banana, peeled
1 cup canned full-fat coconut milk, divided

1. Place watercress, orange, peach, banana, and 1/2 cup coconut milk in a blender and blend until thoroughly combined.
2. Add remaining coconut milk while blending until desired texture is achieved.

Per Serving

Calorie 300| Fat 15g| Carbs 33g| Protein 4g

Classic Strawberry Vanilla Almond Smoothie

Prep time: 15 minutes | Cook time: 0 minutes | Serves 2

1/2 medium banana, peeled and frozen
1/2 cup frozen strawberries
2 tablespoons ground
flaxseed
2 tablespoons rolled oats
1 cup unsweetened vanilla almond milk

1. Place all ingredients in a blender.
2. Purée until smooth.

Per Serving

Calorie 218| Fat 7g| Carbs 35g| Protein 7g

Watercress Mango Smoothie

Prep time: 15 minutes | Cook time: 0 minutes | Serves 2

1 cup chopped watercress
1 medium mango, pitted and peeled
1 cup raspberries
11/2 cups oat milk, divided

1. Place watercress, mango, raspberries, and 3/4 cup oat milk in a blender and blend until thoroughly combined.
2. 2 Add remaining oat milk while blending until desired texture is achieved.

Per Serving

Calorie 232| Fat 3g| Carbs 50g| Protein 6g

CHAPTER 7: DESSERTS, APPETIZERS AND SNACKS

Simple Vegan Brownies

Prep time: 30 minutes | Cook time: 30 minutes | Serves 16

3 Tablespoons ground flaxseed
2/3 cups warm water
1/2 cup coconut flour, sifted
1/2 cup unsweetened cocoa powder
1/2 Teaspoon baking powder
1/4 Teaspoon salt
2/3 cups melted coconut oil
1/2 cup pure maple syrup
1 Tablespoon vanilla extract

1. Preheat the oven to 300°F and lightly grease a square glass baking dish.
2. Whisk together the flaxseed and water in a small bowl – let rest 5 to 10 minutes.
3. Combine the coconut flour, cocoa powder, baking powder and salt in a medium mixing bowl.
4. In another both, whisk together the coconut oil, maple syrup and vanilla extract – whisk in the flaxseed mixture.
5. Whisk the dry ingredients into the wet in small batches until smooth and well combined.
6. Spread the batter in the baking dish and bake for 20 minutes until a knife inserted in the center comes out clean.
7. Cool the brownies completely before cutting into squares to serve.

Per Serving
Calorie 165 | Fats 12g | Carbs 15g | Protein1.5g

Homemade Olive Smoothie

Prep time: 15 minutes | Cook time: 0 minutes | Serves 8

1/2 cup pitted green olives
3/4 cup pitted black olives
2 cloves garlic, peeled
1 tablespoon capers
2 tablespoons lemon juice
2 tablespoons olive oil
1/4 teaspoon oregano
1/4 teaspoon ground black pepper

1. Process all ingredients in a food processor until almost smooth.

Per Serving
Calorie 65 | Fats 7g | Carbs 2g | Protein 0g

World's Best Banana sweet with coconut cream

Prep time: 25 minutes | Cook time: 15 minutes | Serves 4

5 large bananas, peeled
3 Tablespoons pure maple syrup
1/2 to 1 Teaspoon ground cinnamon

1. Preheat the oven to 350°F
2. Grease a small glass baking dish.
3. Slice the bananas and toss them with the maple syrup and cinnamon.
4. Spread the bananas in the baking dish and bake for 15 minutes until tender.
5. Spoon the bananas into bowls and serve with a dollop of coconut cream.

Per Serving
Calorie 190 | Fats 12g | Carbs 49g | Protein 2g

Chocolate Coconut Patties

Prep time: 5 minutes | Cook time: 0 minutes | Serves 24

1/2 cup coconut oil
1 serving liquid sweetener of choice
1/2 cup coconut butter, melted
2 Teaspoons peppermint extract
½ cup cocoa powder

1. With muffin liners and set aside, line a 24-count mini muffin tin.
2. Melt 1 cup of your chocolate chips and evenly distribute between the mini muffin's tins, ensuring the sides are covered in the chocolate. Refrigerate.
3. Slightly melt your coconut butter until smooth and creamy if required. Add your peppermint extract and stir well.
4. Remove the firm chocolate shells and evenly distribute the coconut butter/mint mixture amongst them.
5. Melt the remaining half-cup of chocolate chips and cover the tops of the peppermint patties. Refrigerate until firm.

Per Serving
Calorie 82 | Fats 8g | Carbs 2g | Protein 2g

Vanilla flavoured Fresh Blueberry pie

Prep time: 30 minutes | Cook time: 25 minutes | Serves 6

5 to 6 cups fresh blueberries
1 Tablespoon tapioca starch
1 Teaspoon vanilla extract
1 cup blanched
almond flour
1 Teaspoon ground cinnamon
Pinch salt
1/3 cup coconut oil
1/4 cup chopped almonds

1. Preheat the oven to 375°F and grease a glass pie plate.
2. Toss the blueberries with the tapioca starch and vanilla extract.
3. Spread the blueberries evenly in the pie plate.
4. Combine the almond flour, cinnamon and salt in a mixing bowl – cut in the coconut oil using a fork until it forms a crumbled mixture.
5. Stir in the almonds then spread the mixture over the blueberries.
6. Bake for 20 to 22 minutes until the blueberries are bubbling and the crust is browned.

Per Serving
Calorie 275 | Fats 20g | Carbs 22g | Protein 5g

Super easy and Creamy Sesame Smoothie with Paprika

Prep time: 15 minutes | Cook time: 0 minutes | Serves 20

2 cups sesame seeds
1/2 cup olive oil
1/2 teaspoon paprika

1. Heat oven to 350°F.
2. Spread sesame seeds in a thin layer on a large baking sheet and toast for 5 minutes in the oven, shaking the sheet once to mix. Cool.
3. Process sesame seeds with oil in a food processor or blender until thick and creamy.
4. Garnish with paprika.

Per Serving
Calorie 142 | Fats 15g | Carbs 2g | Protein 3g

Big Fat Dark Chocolate Cookies

Prep time: 22 minute | Cook time: 25 minute | Serves 4

½ cup very dark chocolate chips
½ cup chopped pecans
3-4 large egg whites
1 Teaspoon vanilla
extract
1 ½ cups Stevia
6 Tablespoons unsweetened cocoa powder
¼ Teaspoon salt

1. Heat oven to 350 degrees and Cover the baking sheet in baking parchment and spray with cooking spray.
2. In a mixing bowl, mix stevia, cocoa, salt, chocolate chips, and pecans together.
3. Add vanilla with three egg whites and stir to moisten batter. If all the dry ingredients aren't moistened or it is too thick, add one more egg white. (It should be very soft / sticky, but not soupy.)
4. Place rounded Teaspoons of dough onto the cookie sheet, 2"-3" apart as cookies will spread and thin while baking.
5. Bake for 11-12 minutes.
6. Allow cookies to set-up on the pan for 5-8 minutes before removing to the cooling rack.

Per Serving
Calorie 30 | Fats 2.4g | Carbs 2.4g | Protein 1g

Easy Papaya Mango Avocado Bowl

Prep time: 10 minutes | Cook time: 0 minutes | Serves 4

1 medium papaya, peeled, pitted, and cubed
1 medium mango, peeled, pitted, and cubed
1 medium ripe avocado, pitted, peeled, and diced
1 tablespoon lime juice
2 cups diced, seeded tomato
1/4 cup peeled, diced red onion
2 tablespoons minced fresh cilantro
1 teaspoon finely chopped jalapeño pepper
1 clove garlic, peeled and minced

1. Combine all ingredients in a medium bowl.
2. Mix well and serve.

Per Serving
Calorie 169 | Fats 6g | Carbs 31g | Protein 3g

Epic Eggplant Puree recipe

Prep time: 15 minutes | Cook time: 30 minutes | Serves 10

2 medium eggplants
3 tablespoons olive oil, divided
2 tablespoons lemon juice
1/4 cup tahini
3 cloves garlic, peeled
1/2 teaspoon cumin
1/2 teaspoon chili powder
1/4 teaspoon salt
1 tablespoon chopped fresh parsley

1. Preheat oven to 400°F. Slice eggplants in half lengthwise and prick skin several times with a fork.
2. Place on a large baking sheet, place cut side up and drizzle with 1 tablespoon olive oil.
3. Bake for 30 minutes, or until soft. Allow to cool slightly.
4. Remove inner flesh and place in a medium bowl.
5. Using a large fork or potato masher, mash eggplant together with remaining ingredients until almost smooth.
6. Serve at room temperature.

Per Serving

Calorie 90 | Fats 6g | Carbs 8g | Protein 2g

Garlic Cilantro Spicy Sauce

Prep time: 15 minutes | Cook time: 10 minutes | Serves 12

1/2 cup chopped fresh cilantro
1 1/2 cups chopped tomatoes
1/4 cup chopped sun-dried tomatoes
1/2 cup olive oil
2 teaspoons lime juice
1 teaspoon minced fresh ginger
11/2 teaspoons minced garlic
1 teaspoon minced jalapeño pepper

1. Combine all ingredients in a food processor and pulse quickly to blend. (Salsa should have a slightly chunky texture)

Per Serving

Calorie 87 | Fats 9g | Carbs 2g | Protein 0g

Hot and Spicy Zucchini Sticks

Prep time: 15 minutes | Cook time: 10 minutes | Serves 4

3/4 cup almond flour
1/2 teaspoon garlic powder
3/4 teaspoon Italian seasoning
1/4 teaspoon salt
4 medium zucchini, cut into strips
4 tablespoons olive oil

1. In a large bowl or pan, combine almond flour, garlic powder, Italian seasoning, and salt.
2. Lightly toss zucchini strips with flour mixture, coating well.
3. Heat olive oil in a large skillet or frying pan over medium-high heat. When oil is hot, gently add zucchini strips to pan.
4. Fry until light golden brown on all sides, about 8 minutes.
5. Drain on paper towels. Serve warm.

Per Serving

Calorie 263 | Fats 23g | Carbs 10g | Protein 7g

Mango Tangerines and Cilantro Bowl

Prep time: 15 minutes | Cook time: 0 minutes | Serves 8

1 large mango, peeled, pitted, and chopped
2 medium tangerines, peeled and chopped
1/2 medium red bell pepper, seeded and chopped
1/2 small red onion, peeled and minced
3 cloves garlic, peeled
and minced
1/2 medium jalapeño pepper, seeded and minced
2 tablespoons lime juice
1/2 teaspoon salt
1/4 teaspoon ground black pepper
3 tablespoons chopped fresh cilantro

1. Gently toss together all ingredients in a large bowl.
2. Allow to sit for at least 15 minutes before serving to allow flavors to mingle.

Per Serving

Calorie 43 | Fats 0g | Carbs 11g | Protein 1g

Restaurant style Spicy Salsa

Prep time: 15 minutes | Cook time: 30 minutes | Serves 16

1/2 pound fresh tomatillos, husked and coarsely chopped
1/2 pound Roma tomatoes, coarsely chopped
1 medium zucchini, coarsely chopped
2 tablespoons olive oil
1 medium onion, peeled and chopped
2 small jalapeño peppers, seeded and chopped
4 cloves garlic, peeled and chopped
2 tablespoons lemon juice
1/2 teaspoon salt
1/8 teaspoon ground black pepper
1/2 teaspoon crushed red pepper flakes
2 tablespoons chopped fresh cilantro

1. Preheat oven to 400°F. Place tomatillos, tomatoes, and zucchini on a large rimmed baking sheet.
2. Drizzle with olive oil and stir to coat. Top with onion.
3. Roast for 20–25 minutes or until vegetables are soft and light brown on the edges.
4. Remove from oven and place in large bowl.
5. Stir in jalapeño peppers, garlic, lemon juice, salt, black pepper, red pepper flakes, and cilantro.
6. Cool, then store in refrigerator for up to one week.

Per Serving
Calorie 30 | Fats 2g | Carbs 3g | Protein 1g

Chef's favorite Classic Avocado salad

Prep time: 15 minutes | Cook time: 10 minutes | Serves 4

2 large ripe avocados, pitted, peeled, and coarsely chopped
1 small white onion, peeled and diced
1 medium tomato, diced
1 medium jalapeño pepper, seeded and thinly sliced
Juice of 1 medium lime

1. Gently combine all ingredients in a small serving bowl and serve as a salad or dip.

Per Serving
Calorie 129 | Fats 11g | Carbs 10g | Protein 2g

Super Tasty Five Pepper Salsa

Prep time: 15 minutes | Cook time: 10 minutes | Serves 8

1 medium yellow bell pepper, seeded and chopped
1 medium orange bell pepper, seeded and chopped
2 small poblano chili peppers, seeded and chopped
2 small Anaheim chili peppers, seeded and chopped
2 medium jalapeño peppers, seeded and chopped
2 cloves garlic, peeled
1/4 medium red onion, peeled
Juice of 1/2 medium lime
1 teaspoon ground black pepper
2 tablespoons olive oil
1 (15-ounce) can black beans, rinsed and drained
1/4 cup chopped cilantro

1. Place peppers, garlic, onion, lime juice, and black pepper in a food processor and pulse until slightly chunky.
2. In a medium saucepan, heat olive oil over medium-high heat until slightly smoking. Add pepper mixture and black beans.
3. Cook for 8–10 minutes, stirring occasionally.
4. Remove from heat and sprinkle with cilantro. Serve hot, cold, or at room temperature.

Per Serving
Calorie 109 | Fats 4g | Carbs 15g | Protein 4g

Delicious Cinnamon Jonathan Apples

Prep time: 15 minutes | Cook time: 30 minutes | Serves 6

3 pounds Jonathan apples, peeled, cored, and coarsely chopped
1/2 cup water
1/2 cup maple syrup
1/2 teaspoon ground cinnamon

1. Combine all ingredients except cinnamon in a 6-quart slow cooker and cover.
2. Cook on high until apples are very soft, about 30 minutes.
3. Sprinkle with cinnamon just before serving.

Per Serving
Calorie 186 | Fats 0g | Carbs 49g | Protein 2g

Indian spiced Crispy Kale Chips

Prep time: 15 minutes | Cook time: 10 minutes | Serves 6

2 large bunches of kale
2 tablespoons extra-virgin olive oil
1 tablespoon coconut oil, melted
2 tablespoons curry powder
1 teaspoon ground ginger
1/2 teaspoon ground cardamom
1/4 teaspoon cayenne pepper
1 teaspoon salt

1. Preheat oven to 350°F. Wash kale well and dry thoroughly. Cut out any large ribs and discard. Cut kale leaves into 3" pieces.
2. In a small bowl, combine olive oil and coconut oil and mix well. Stir in curry powder, ginger, cardamom, and cayenne pepper and mix until combined.
3. Pour curry mixture over kale leaves and massage with your hands until the leaves are coated.
4. Arrange leaves in a single layer on two large baking sheets. Bake for 15–18 minutes, rotating pans after 10 minutes.
5. Remove from oven and sprinkle with salt. Let stand until leaves are crisp.
6. Store at room temperature in airtight container for up to one week.

Per Serving
Calorie 79 | Fats 7g | Carbs 4g | Protein 1g

Homemade Instant Roasted Pistachios

Prep time: 15 minutes | Cook time: 0 minutes | Serves 16

1 pound raw pistachios
2 tablespoons extra-virgin olive oil

1. Add nuts and olive oil to a 2-quart slow cooker.
2. Stir to combine. Cover and cook on low for 20 minutes.
3. Stir mixture again and Cover and cook for 10 more minutes.
4. Cool and store in an airtight container in the refrigerator for up to several months.

Per Serving
Calorie 173 | Fats 15g | Carbs 8g | Protein 6g

Apricot Date Baby Puree

Prep time: 15 minutes | Cook time: 15 minutes | Serves 4

6 medium apples, peeled, cored, and chopped
1/3 cup water
1/2 cup chopped
dried apricots
4 large pitted dates, chopped
1/4 teaspoon ground cinnamon

1. Add apples and water to a large soup pot or stockpot and brings to a low boil over medium-high heat.
2. Reduce heat to low, cover, and simmer for 15 minutes, stirring occasionally.
3. Add apricots and dates and simmer for another 10–15 minutes.
4. Mash with a large fork until desired consistency is reached, or allow cooling slightly and purée in a blender until smooth.
5. Sprinkle with cinnamon before serving.

Per Serving
Calorie 213 | Fats 1g | Carbs 57g | Protein 2g

Cinnamon spiced roasted Walnuts

Prep time: 15 minutes | Cook time: 30 minutes | Serves 6

11/2 cups walnuts
1/4 cup maple syrup
2 teaspoons cinnamon
11/2 teaspoons chili powder
2 teaspoons coconut oil

1. Combine all ingredients in a greased (with olive oil) 21/2-quart slow cooker.
2. Cover slow cooker and vent lid with a chopstick or the handle of a wooden spoon.
3. Cook on high for15 minutes.
4. If using a larger slow cooker, you will probably need to reduce the cooking time to only 15 minutes.
5. Line a large baking sheet with parchment paper.
6. Pour walnut mixture onto the baking sheet and spread out into one layer.
7. Allow to cool and dry and then transfer to a container with an airtight lid.
8. Store in the pantry for up to two weeks

Per Serving
Calorie 211 | Fats 18g | Carbs 49g | Protein 1g

Chilled Tomato salad with Melon

Prep time: 15 minutes | Cook time: 0 minutes | Serves 4

3 large tomatoes, seeded and finely diced
1/2 large honeydew melon, peeled, seeded, and diced
1 medium cantaloupe, peeled, seeded, and diced
1 cup peeled, diced red onion
1 small jalapeño pepper, seeded and minced
1/2 cup chopped fresh cilantro
Juice of 1 large lime

1. In a large serving bowl, combine all ingredients and mix well.
2. Chill for 4 hours before serving.

Per Serving

Calorie 152 | Fats 1g | Carbs 37g | Protein 4g

Magical Dried Fruit and Nut curry

Prep time: 15 minutes | Cook time: 10 minutes | Serves 16

1 cup broken walnuts
1 cup small whole pecans
2 tablespoons coconut oil
1 tablespoon extra-virgin olive oil
1 tablespoon curry powder
1 cup sunflower seeds
1 cup unsweetened dried cranberries
1/2 cup chopped dried unsulfured apricots

1. In a medium bowl, combine walnuts and pecans; set aside.
2. In a large saucepan, combine coconut oil and olive oil; melt over medium heat.
3. Add curry powder; cook and stir for about 1 minute until fragrant.
4. Add walnuts and pecans to saucepan; cook, stirring frequently, until nuts are toasted and slightly crisp.
5. Remove walnuts and pecans from heat and transfer nuts back to bowl.
6. Add sunflower seeds to pan and toast for 1–2 minutes. Add to bowl.
7. Stir in cranberries and apricots and toss to coat.
8. Spread on paper towel and let cool.
9. Store in an airtight container for up to several days.

Per Serving

Calorie 183 | Fats 15g | Carbs 12g | Protein 3g

Mushroom and Vegetables with Pepper

Prep time: 15 minutes | Cook time: 10 minutes | Serves 6

6 wooden skewers, cut in half and soaked in water for at least 1 hour
12 green onions, trimmed
1 large red bell pepper, seeded and cut into large chunks
1 large yellow bell pepper, seeded and cut into large chunks
1 large green bell pepper, seeded and cut into large chunks
12 large button mushrooms
1 tablespoon olive oil
1/2 tablespoon ground black pepper

1. Preheat grill or broiler.
2. Thread vegetables onto skewers, and brush all sides of vegetables with oil. Season with pepper.
3. Place skewers on the grill or under the broiler, paying close attention as they cook, as they can easily burn.
4. Cook about 10 minutes, until vegetables are fork tender.

Per Serving

Calorie 60 | Fats 3g | Carbs 8g | Protein 2g

Olive Oil Roasted Almonds

Prep time: 15 minutes | Cook time: 30 minutes | Serves 10

21/2 cups skin-on almonds
1 teaspoon olive oil
1/2 teaspoon ground jalapeño
1/2 teaspoon garlic powder
1/2 teaspoon cayenne pepper
1/2 teaspoon ground chipotle
1/2 teaspoon ground paprika

1. Place nuts in a 2–4-quart slow cooker. Drizzle with olive oil and Stir.
2. Add remaining ingredients and stir again to distribute seasonings evenly.
3. Cover slow cooker and cook on high for 20 minutes.
4. Uncover and cook on low for 10 minutes or until nuts look dry.
5. Store in an airtight container in the refrigerator for up to several months.

Per Serving

Calorie 176 | Fats 16g | Carbs 6g | Protein 6g

Dark Chocolate Nut Clusters

Prep time: 15 minutes | Cook time: 15 minutes | Serves 16

1 cup hazelnuts
1 cup walnuts
11/2 cups pecans

1 pound dark chocolate, cut into small pieces

1. Preheat oven to 350°F. Place hazelnuts, walnuts, and pecans on a large baking sheet.
2. Bake for 10–15 minutes or just until nuts are fragrant and start to brown. Remove from oven and cool completely.
3. Coarsely chop nuts and place on a parchment paper–lined baking sheet.
4. Reserve 1/3 cup chocolate; place the remaining chocolate in a small, heavy saucepan over low heat.
5. Melt, stirring occasionally, until mixture is smooth. Remove from heat and stir in reserved chocolate until melted; this tempers the chocolate so it will stay solid at room temperature.
6. Pour chocolate over nuts to coat. Let stand until set, then break into bars. Store in airtight container at room temperature for up to one week

Per Serving
Calorie 307 | Fats 24g | Carbs 21g | Protein 4g

Watermelon Coconut milk Pops

Prep time: 15 minutes | Cook time: 0 minutes | Makes 8 pops

2 cups cubed seedless watermelon
1/2 cup canned full-fat coconut milk

1 tablespoon lime juice
1 tablespoon maple syrup

1. Combine all ingredients in blender or food processor and blend or process until smooth.
2. Pour into frozen-pop molds and insert sticks. If using paper cups or muffin tins, freeze for about an hour, and then insert sticks.
3. Cover and freeze until firm, about 5–7 hours. Unmold to serve.

Per Serving
Calorie 40 | Fats 2g | Carbs 5g | Protein 1g

Garlic Pepper Pumpkin Seed Roast

Prep time: 15 minutes | Cook time: 15 minutes | Serves 12

3 cups raw pumpkin seeds
1/2 cup olive oil
1/2 teaspoon garlic

powder
1/2 teaspoon ground black pepper

1. Preheat oven to 300°F.
2. In a medium bowl, mix together all ingredients until pumpkin seeds are evenly coated.
3. Spread in an even layer on a large baking sheet.
4. Bake for 30 and stirring every 10–15 minutes.
5. Store in an airtight container for up to several months.

Per Serving
Calorie 249 | Fats 24g | Carbs 4g | Protein 9g

Super Tasty Ginger Garlic Walnuts

Prep time: 15 minutes | Cook time: 30 minutes | Serves 12

2 tablespoons coconut oil
1/4 cup maple syrup
1 teaspoon ground ginger
1 teaspoon curry powder

1/2 teaspoon cayenne
1/4 teaspoon onion powder
1/4 teaspoon garlic powder
3 cups shelled walnuts

1. Place coconut oil in a 2–4-quart slow cooker, turn on high, and allow oil to melt.
2. While oil is melting, mix maple syrup, ginger, curry powder, cayenne, onion powder, and garlic powder together in a small bowl.
3. Once oil has melted, add walnuts to slow cooker and stir.
4. Add maple syrup mixture to slow cooker, and stir until nuts are evenly coated.
5. Cover and cook on high for 15 minutes.
6. Remove cover and cook for an additional 15 minutes, until nuts are dry.
7. Cool and store in airtight containers in a cool, dry place for up to several weeks

Per Serving
Calorie 202 | Fats 19g | Carbs 8g | Protein 4g

Spicy Garlic Roasted Almonds

Prep time: 15 minutes | Cook time: 30 minutes | Serves 24

6 cups whole raw almonds
4 tablespoons coconut oil
3 cloves garlic, peeled and minced
2 teaspoons coarsely ground black pepper

1. Heat a 4-quart slow cooker on high for 15 minutes.
2. Add almonds. Drizzle oil over almonds and stir.
3. Sprinkle with garlic and black pepper and stir.
4. Cover and cook on low 15 minutes, stirring every 5 minutes.
5. Turn heat up to high and cook uncovered for 2 minutes
6. Turn heat to low and serve warm or remove from heat and allow cooling.
7. Store in an airtight container in the refrigerator for up to several months.

Per Serving

Calorie 190 | Fats 17g | Carbs 6g | Protein 6g

Easy Roasted Pumpkin Seeds

Prep time: 15 minutes | Cook time: 25 minutes | Serves 16

2 cups pumpkin seeds
1 tablespoon grass-fed butter, melted
2 tablespoons coconut sugar
2 teaspoons cinnamon
1/2 teaspoon salt
1/4 teaspoon nutmeg

1. Preheat oven to 325°F. Place pumpkin seeds on a large rimmed baking sheet.
2. Drizzle with butter and stir to coat.
3. Spread into a single layer. Sprinkle with coconut sugar.
4. Roast for 18–23 minutes, stirring once during cooking, until seeds are light golden brown.
5. Sprinkle with cinnamon, salt, and nutmeg and toss to coat.
6. Cool completely before storing in an airtight container for up to one week.

Per Serving

Calorie 97| Fats 8g | Carbs 4g | Protein 4g

Cayenne Pepper Roasted Cashews with Honey

Prep time: 15 minutes | Cook time: 30 minutes | Serves 24

6 cups cashews
3 tablespoons olive oil
3 tablespoons crushed dried rosemary leaves
1 tablespoon honey
3/4 teaspoon cayenne pepper
1/2 teaspoon garlic powder

1. Heat a 2–4-quart slow cooker on high for 15 minutes
2. Add cashews. Drizzle olive oil over cashews and toss to coat.
3. Add remaining ingredients and stir to combine.
4. Cover and cook on low for 15 minutes.
5. Turn heat to high, uncover, and cook for 10 minutes, stirring after 5 minutes.
6. Turn heat to low to keep warm for serving or remove from slow cooker and Store in an airtight container in the refrigerator for up to several months

Per Serving

Calorie 199 | Fats 16g | Carbs 11g | Protein 6g

Grandma's Special Caramel-Nuts Mix

Prep time: 15 minutes | Cook time: 30 minutes | Serves 16

4 cups mixed raw almonds, pecan and walnut halves
1/2 cup
"Butterscotch-Caramel" Sauce
11/2 teaspoons cinnamon

1. Add all ingredients to a 1-quart slow cooker.
2. Stir to coat nuts. Cover and cook on low for 20 minutes, stirring at least once in 10 minutes.
3. Uncover slow cooker. Stirring mixture every 5 minutes or until it is almost dry.
4. Line a large baking sheet with parchment paper. Evenly spread nuts on the sheet and allow cooling completely.
5. Store in a covered container at room temperature for up to several weeks

Per Serving

Calorie 244 | Fats 20g | Carbs 14g | Protein 6g

Perfectly Roasted Parsnip Chips

Prep time: 15 minutes | Cook time: 30 minutes | Serves 6

6 large parsnips, peeled and cut diagonally into thin slices

3 tablespoons olive oil
1/8 teaspoon nutmeg
1 teaspoon cinnamon

1. Preheat oven to 400°F. Spray a large baking sheet with cooking spray.
2. In a large bowl, combine parsnips, olive oil, and spices and stir to coat.
3. Arrange parsnips on baking sheet in a single layer and cook for 25 minutes.
4. Remove from oven and turn on broiler.
5. Broil chips for 5 minutes.
6. Serve warm or at room temperature.

Per Serving

Calorie 177 | Fats 7g | Carbs 28g | Protein 2g

Vanilla flavoured Berry Mix Bowl

Prep time: 5 minutes | Cook time: 0 minutes | Serves 2

1 (14-ounce) can full-fat coconut milk, chilled
½ teaspoon alcohol-free vanilla extract
2 cups fresh berries (blueberries,

strawberries, raspberries, blackberries, or a mixture)
2 tablespoons chopped fresh mint, for garnish (optional)

1. Open the can of coconut milk without shaking it and scoop out the thickened coconut cream from the top into a medium bowl, reserving the water for drinking or a smoothie.
2. Add the vanilla and whisk until thickened.
3. To serve, divide half of the berries between two chilled beverage glasses.
4. Top with about 2 inches of the cream.
5. Add the remaining berries and top with the remaining cream.
6. Garnish with the mint (if using) and serve.

Per Serving

Calorie 503 | Fats 48g | Carbs 22g | Protein 6g

Mulberry-Pistachio Salad

Prep time: 15 minutes | Cook time: 10 minutes | Serves 12

1/2 cup pistachio nuts
1/2 cup pumpkin seeds
1/2 cup sunflower seeds

1/2 cup unsweetened coconut flakes
1 cup dried mulberries

1. Combine all ingredients in a medium bowl. S
2. Serve immediately or store in an airtight container at room temperature for up to one week.

Per Serving

Calorie 140 | Fats 10g | Carbs 10g | Protein 5g

Homemade-Coconut Oil Baked Seeds Mix

Prep time: 10 minutes | Cook time: 30 minutes | Serves 6

¾ cup sesame seeds
⅓ cup sunflower seeds
¼ cup chia seeds
3 tablespoons pepitas (pumpkin seeds)

2 tablespoons flaxseeds
1 ⅔ cups water
1 teaspoon salt
3 tablespoons coconut oil, melted

1. Preheat the oven to 350°F.
2. In a large bowl, combine the seeds with the water and let them soak until they have absorbed the liquid and a thick dough forms, about 20 minutes.
3. Add the salt and stir well to combine.
4. Lightly grease a baking sheet with 1 tablespoon of the melted coconut oil.
5. Using a rubber spatula or wooden spoon, spread the dough in a thin layer (¼ inch or less) on the baking sheet.
6. Brush the top with the remaining 2 tablespoons coconut oil and bake until set and slightly browned on one side.
7. Remove the baking sheet from the oven.
8. Cool enough to handle, carefully break the cracker into smaller pieces.

Per Serving

Calorie 262 | Fats 23g | Carbs 10g | Protein 7g

Pecan and Walnut Holiday Nut Mix

Prep time: 15 minutes | Cook time: 30 minutes | Serves 24

2 large eggs
1 teaspoon lemon juice
1/4 teaspoon salt
2 tablespoons maple syrup
11/2 teaspoons cinnamon
1 teaspoon chili powder
1/2 teaspoon cayenne

pepper
1/2 cup finely chopped coconut
2 cups walnuts
2 cups pecans
2 cups hazelnuts
1/4 cup extra-virgin olive oil
3 tablespoons coconut oil, melted

1. Preheat oven to 325°F. In a large bowl, beat eggs with lemon juice and salt until stiff peaks form.
2. Beat in maple syrup, cinnamon, chili powder, and cayenne pepper until combined. Stir in coconut.
3. Fold in walnuts, pecans, and hazelnuts until nuts are coated.
4. Spread olive oil and coconut oil in 15" × 10" jellyroll pan.
5. Spread nuts over oil mixture.
6. Bake for 20 minutes, stirring every 10 minutes, until nuts are light golden brown and crisp and oil is absorbed.
7. Let cool, then store in an airtight container at room temperature for up to several days.

Per Serving
Calorie 236 | Fats 23g | Carbs 6g | Protein 4g

Sweet and Spicy Cashew Almond Mix

Prep time: 15 minutes | Cook time: 25 minutes | Serves 8

1/2 cup cashews
1/2 cup almonds
1/2 cup macadamia nuts
1/2 cup pistachio nuts
4 tablespoons honey
1 teaspoon sea salt
1/2 teaspoon ground black pepper

1/4 teaspoon ground cumin
1 teaspoon curry powder
1/8 teaspoon ground cloves
1 teaspoon ground cinnamon

1. Preheat oven to 300°F. and Place cashews, almonds, macadamias, and pistachios on a large baking sheet and bake for 10–12 minutes, taking care they do not burn.
2. Remove from oven and let cool approximately 5 minutes.
3. In a small bowl, mix honey, salt, pepper, cumin; curry powder, cloves, and cinnamon.
4. In a large saucepan over medium heat, place nuts and half the honey mixture. When mixture begins to melt, mix in remaining honey mixture.
5. Shake the pan and stir until nuts are coated, about 5 minutes.
6. Remove nuts from the pan and spread them out on a sheet of parchment paper. Use a spoon to separate nuts that stick together.
7. Let dry for about 30 minutes

Per Serving
Calorie 223 | Fats 17g | Carbs 16g | Protein 5g

Ghee roasted Almond Pecan Mix

Prep time: 15 minutes | Cook time: 30 minutes | Serves 24

4 tablespoons ghee
3 tablespoons lime juice
2 teaspoons garlic powder
2 teaspoons onion powder
1 cup raw almonds

1 cup raw pecans
1 cup raw walnut pieces
1 cup raw cashews
2 cups raw pumpkin seeds, shelled
1 cup raw sunflower seeds, shelled

1. Add ghee to a 2-quart slow cooker. Then add lime juice, garlic powder, and onion powder, and stir all together.
2. Add remaining ingredients and stir well until nuts and seeds are evenly coated. Cover and cook on low for 25 minutes, stirring occasionally.
3. Uncover slow cooker, stir, and cook for another 5 minute, to dry nuts and seeds.
4. Cool and store in airtight container for up to several weeks

Per Serving
Calorie 231 | Fats 21g | Carbs 7g | Protein 7g

Lemony Dates with Hazelnuts

Prep time: 15 minutes | Cook time: 30 minutes | Serves 8

2 cups pitted dates, soaked in water overnight
2/3 cup boiling water
1/4 cup maple syrup

Strips of peel from 1 medium lemon (yellow part only)
1/4 cup hazelnuts

1. Preheat oven to 350°F. Spread hazelnuts on a baking sheet and bake for 8–10 minutes.
2. Drain dates and place in a 41/2-quart slow cooker.
3. Add boiling water, maple syrup, and lemon peel. Cover and cook on high for 20 minutes.
4. Discard lemon peel. Place dates on a serving dish and sprinkle with hazelnuts.

Per Serving

Calorie 135 | Fats 3g | Carbs 29g | Protein 1g

Tasty Cashew Pepper Cheese dip

Prep time: 5 minutes | Cook time: 0 minutes | Serves 2

1 cup raw cashews
2 teaspoons lemon juice
¼ teaspoon salt
¼ teaspoons freshly

ground black pepper
3 tablespoons cold water, plus more as needed

1. Soak the cashews in a bowl of water to cover for at least 1 hour and up to overnight in the refrigerator.
2. Drain, briefly rinse, and transfer the cashews to a food processor.
3. Add the lemon juice, salt, and pepper and pulse until combined, about 1 minute.
4. Scrape down the sides of the food processor with a rubber spatula, add the water, and process until smooth, 2 to 4 minutes, adding more water by the teaspoon to thin it out if needed.
5. Add optional dip flavors and process until combined.
6. Serve with Gluten-Free Seedy Crackers.

Per Serving

Calorie 351 | Fats 26g | Carbs 17g | Protein 11g

Salty Brown Apple

Prep time: 7 minutes | Cook time: 30 minutes | Serves 4

2 apples, cored

¼ teaspoon salt

1. Preheat the oven to 275°F. Line a baking sheet with aluminium foil or parchment paper.
2. Using a mandolin or sharp knife, thinly slice the apples. Spread them out flat on the prepared baking sheet in an even layer.
3. Sprinkle evenly with the salt and, if desired, other spices
4. Bake until crisp on one side, about 20 minutes, Turn the slices over and bake until completely crisped and lightly browned.
5. Remove from the oven and allow cooling before storing.

Per Serving

Calorie 58 | Fats 0g | Carbs 15g | Protein 0g

Chocolate flavoured Almond Ball

Prep time: 5 minutes | Cook time: 10 minutes | Serves 16

1½ cups raw almonds
½ cup creamy unsalted almond butter
¼ cup raw cacao powder

3 tablespoons coconut oil, melted
2 tablespoons raw honey or maple syrup
¼ teaspoon ground cinnamon

1. Place the nuts in a food processor and pulse until finely ground.
2. Add the remaining ingredients and pulse until a smooth, sticky dough forms, 1 to 2 minutes.
3. Scoop out 1 heaping tablespoon of dough at a time to form 1½-inch balls, placing them on an aluminum foil– or parchment paper–lined baking sheet or plate so they don't touch.
4. Refrigerate the truffles until firm, about 1 hour.

Per Serving

Calorie 148 | Fats 12g | Carbs 7g | Protein 5g

Golden Hazelnut Crackers

Prep time: 15 minutes | Cook time: 15 minutes | Makes 30 crackers

1 cup hazelnut flour
3/4 cup coconut flour
1/4 cup tapioca starch
1/4 teaspoon baking soda
1/2 teaspoon cream of tartar
2 teaspoons cinnamon
1/4 teaspoon salt
1/3 cup maple syrup
3 tablespoons coconut oil
1/4 cup canned full-fat coconut milk
1 tablespoon water
2 teaspoons vanilla

1. Preheat oven to 350°F. In a large bowl, combine hazelnut flour, coconut flour, tapioca starch, baking soda, cream of tartar, cinnamon, and salt, and mix until one color.
2. In a small saucepan, combine maple syrup, coconut oil, coconut milk, and water and heat until oil melts.
3. Add coconut milk mixture to dry ingredients along with vanilla, and mix until dough forms.
4. Line a baking sheet with parchment paper. Roll dough into 2" balls and place on lined baking sheet about 3" apart.
5. Top with another sheet of parchment paper and flatten balls using a rolling pin to 1/8" thickness.
6. Carefully peel off the top piece of paper. Prick the dough with a fork.
7. Bake for 12–15 minutes or until crackers are set and golden brown.

Per Serving
Calorie 127 | Fats 9g | Carbs 11g | Protein 2g

Chilled Peach Chocolate Pops

Prep time: 5 minutes | Cook time: 0 minutes | Serves 10

12 tablespoons raw cacao powder
6 tablespoons fresh peach purée
6 tablespoons coconut oil
6 tablespoons canned full-fat coconut milk
3 tablespoons unsweetened shredded coconut
2 tablespoons cacao nibs
1 medium ripe banana

1. Combine all ingredients in a food processor and pulse until very smooth. Add water if the consistency is not fluid.
2. Pour into ice cube trays and freeze for at least 6 hours.

Chilled Coconut Banana Dessert

Prep time: 4 minutes | Cook time: 0 minutes | Serves 4

4 bananas, peeled and sliced into 2-inch pieces
¼ cup unsweetened
flaked coconut
¼ cup coconut milk
2 tablespoons almond butter

1. Freeze the bananas for at least an hour or overnight.
2. Add the bananas to a food processor or blender. Pulse a few times to break down.
3. Add the flaked coconut, coconut milk, and almond butter and process until smooth, 3 to 4 minutes.
4. Scrape down the sides of the food processor and serve immediately in chilled bowls or freeze for later enjoyment.

Per Serving
Calorie 412 | Fats 20g | Carbs 60g | Protein 7g

Almond Strawberry Pumpkin Salad

Prep time: 15 minutes | Cook time: 10 minutes | Serves 16

1 cup raw almonds
1 cup pumpkin seeds
1/2 cup sunflower seeds
1 cup dehydrated strawberries
1/2 cup goji berries

1. Combine all ingredients in a medium bowl.
2. Serve immediately or store in an airtight container at room temperature for up to one week.

Per Serving
Calorie 139 | Fats 10g | Carbs 7g | Protein 5g

Macadamia Snack with Egg fills and Raspberry Sauce

Prep time: 10 minutes | Cook time: 20 minutes | Makes 12 triangles

For Crust
3 cups raw macadamia nuts
½ cup coconut oil, melted
¼ teaspoon ground cinnamon
For filling
4 large eggs, at room temperature
3 tablespoons grated
lemon zest (from 3 to 4 lemons)
½ cup lemon juice (from about 4 lemons)
½ cup coconut oil
2 tablespoons maple syrup
1 teaspoon alcohol-free vanilla extract

For sauce
1 cup fresh raspberries
1 teaspoon water

1. Preheat the oven to 350°F.
2. To make the crust, into a food processor put the nuts, coconut oil, and cinnamon and pulse until slightly chunky but sticky and dough-like.
3. Into the bottom of a 9-inch round tart pan, pie plate, or spring form pan, press the crust mixture.
4. Bake until the crust is set and slightly golden, about 10 minutes. Remove it from the oven and let it cool.
5. To make the filling, in a medium bowl beat the eggs; set aside.
6. Into a small saucepan put the lemon zest and juice, coconut oil, maple syrup, and vanilla and whisk to combine. Heat over medium heat until warm.
7. Spoon a few tablespoons of the heated mixture into the eggs, whisking constantly to temper the eggs.
8. Add the egg mixture to the saucepan, reduce the heat to medium-low, and cook until thickened, whisking constantly.
9. Pour the lemon filling into the crust, spreading it with a rubber spatula or wooden spoon into an even layer.
10. Refrigerate until firmly set (it shouldn't jiggle when you shake it), about 1 hour.
11. Meanwhile, make the sauce. In a saucepan, heat the raspberries and water over medium heat, whisking until smooth with some chunks.
12. Heat until warmed through and slightly thickened.
13. To serve, cut the tart into quarters and then cut each quarter into three small triangles.
14. Top with the raspberry sauce.

Per Serving
Calorie 190 | Fats 12g | Carbs 49g | Protein 2g

Healthy Date Coconut Flake Cookies

Prep time: 5 minutes | Cook time: 15 minutes | Serves 12

1 cup chopped pitted dates
1 medium banana, peeled
1/4 teaspoon vanilla
13/4 cups unsweetened coconut flakes

1. Preheat oven to 375°F. Cover dates in water and soak for about 10 minutes until softened. Drain.
2. Process together dates, banana, and vanilla in a food processor until almost smooth. Stir in coconut flakes by hand until thick. You may need a little more or less than 13/4 cups.
3. Drop by generous tablespoonful onto a cookie sheet.
4. Bake for 10–12 minutes or until golden brown. Cookies will be soft and chewy.

Cinnamon Nutty Fruity Dessert

Prep time: 5 minutes | Cook time: 30 minutes | Serves 6

4 cups peeled, cored, sliced apples
1/2 cup sliced cranberries
1/3 cup maple syrup
2 tablespoons coconut oil
1 teaspoon ground cinnamon
1/4 teaspoon ground nutmeg
3/4 cup combined chopped walnuts and almonds

1. Combine all ingredients except nuts in a cooker.
2. Cover and cook on high for 30 minutes or until apples are tender.
3. Sprinkle each serving with nuts.

Walnut Coconut Chocolate Squares

Prep time: 5 minutes | Cook time: 0 minutes | Serves 16

1 cup finely chopped walnuts
1 cup unsweetened grated coconut
3 cups crushed "Graham" Crackers
2/3 cup canned full-fat coconut milk
14 ounces chopped dark chocolate
2 teaspoons vanilla

1. Grease a 9" square pan with coconut oil and set aside.
2. In a large bowl, combine walnuts, coconut, and cracker crumbs; set aside.
3. In medium saucepan, combine coconut milk and chocolate.
4. Melt over low heat, stirring frequently, until smooth. Stir in vanilla. Reserve 1/3 cup of this mixture.
5. Pour remaining chocolate mixture over crumb mixture and stir to coat.
6. Press crumb mixture into prepared pan and spread reserved chocolate over top.
7. Place in refrigerator until set; cut into eight squares to serve.

Raisin Walnut Cookies

Prep time: 5 minutes | Cook time: 15 minutes | Makes 48 squares

2 cups maple syrup
4 cups almond flour
1/2 teaspoon nutmeg
1/2 teaspoon ginger
1/2 cup dates,
chopped
2 cups ground walnuts
1/2 cup raisins

1. Preheat oven to 350°F. Line two large baking sheets with parchment paper.
2. Warm maple syrup in a medium saucepan over low heat for 5 minutes and let cool slightly.
3. In a medium bowl, sift together flour, nutmeg, and ginger.
4. Add maple syrup and stir until well blended. Stir in dates, walnuts, and raisins.
5. Roll dough to 1/4" thick and cut into forty-eight squares.
6. Place squares on prepared baking sheets and bake for 10 minutes.
7. Remove and cool.

Walnut Currant Apple

Prep time: 5 minutes | Cook time: 30 minutes | Serves 4

1/4 cup coarsely chopped walnuts
3 tablespoons dried currants
3/4 teaspoon ground
cinnamon, divided
4 medium Granny Smith apples, cored
1 cup maple syrup
3/4 cup apple cider

1. In a small bowl, combine walnuts and currants.
2. Add 1/4 teaspoon cinnamon, stirring to combine.
3. Place apples in a cooker.
4. Spoon walnut mixture into the cavity of each apple.
5. In a medium mixing bowl, combine remaining 1/2 teaspoon cinnamon, maple syrup, and apple cider, stirring to combine.
6. Pour over apples in the cooker.
7. Cover and cook for 30 minutes.
8. Remove apples with a slotted spoon.
9. Spoon 1/4 cup cooking liquid over each serving.

Banana Muffins with Cocoa Nibs

Prep time: 5 minutes | Cook time: 30 minutes | Serves 4

4 small bananas, peeled
1/2 teaspoon grated orange rind
1/2 tablespoon pear purée
1 tablespoon lemon juice
1/8 teaspoon cinnamon
1/8 teaspoon nutmeg
1 tablespoon coconut oil, melted
1 tablespoon cacao nibs

1. Preheat oven to 350°F.
2. Cut each banana lengthwise and across into eight pieces. Arrange banana slices in a small baking pan.
3. Sprinkle evenly with orange rind, pear purée, lemon juice, cinnamon, nutmeg, and coconut oil.
4. Bake uncovered for 25-30 minutes, basting after 5 minutes with liquid in baking pan.
5. Sprinkle with cacao nibs before serving.

No sugar Orange Juice Apple Pie

Prep time: 15 minutes | Cook time: 30 minutes | Serves 8

8 medium apples, peeled, cored, and sliced
3 tablespoons orange juice
3 tablespoons water
1/2 cup chopped

pecans
1/3 cup maple syrup
1/4 cup grass-fed butter, melted
1/2 teaspoon cinnamon

1. Grease a cooker with olive oil.
2. Arrange apple slices to cover the bottom of the cooker.
3. In a small bowl or measuring cup, stir orange juice and water to mix. Evenly drizzle over apples.
4. In another small bowl, combine pecans, maple syrup, butter, and cinnamon; mix well.
5. Evenly crumble pecan mixture over apples.
6. Cover and cook for 30 minutes.
7. Serve warm or chilled

Nutty Fruity Pies

Prep time: 5 minutes | Cook time: 30 minutes | Serves 6

1/2 cup oat flour
1/4 cup almond flour
1/2 cup chopped toasted hazelnuts
1/4 cup shredded coconut
1/3 cup coconut oil, melted
2 tablespoons maple syrup, divided

1/4 teaspoon salt
3 medium ripe peaches, peeled and chopped
1 cup blueberries
1 cup raspberries
1 teaspoon vanilla
1 tablespoon orange juice

1. Preheat oven to 400°F. Grease six (1-cup) ovenproof custard cups with coconut oil and set aside.
2. In a medium bowl, combine oat flour, almond flour, hazelnuts, and coconut and toss.
3. Add melted coconut oil, 1 tablespoon maple syrup, and salt and mix until crumbly; set aside.
4. In another medium bowl, combine peaches, blueberries, and raspberries.

5. Sprinkle with vanilla, orange juice and remaining 1 tablespoon maple syrup and toss gently.
6. Divide among prepared custard cups. Top with crumble mixture.
7. Place custard cups on a large rimmed baking sheet and bake for 20–30 minutes or until fruit is bubbly and tender and topping is browned.
8. Serve warm or cool.

Maple Pineapple with Macadamia Nuts

Prep time: 5 minutes | Cook time: 10 minutes | Serves 6

1 large pineapple, cored, peeled, and cut into 1" rings
1/4 cup maple syrup

2 tablespoons finely chopped macadamia nuts

1. Coat grill rack with non-stick cooking spray and preheat grill.
2. Grill pineapple over medium heat for 5 minutes. Turn pineapple over and grill 5 more minutes.
3. Remove pineapple from grill and place on a serving platter.
4. Brush with maple syrup and sprinkle with macadamia nuts.

Easy Cranberry Pears Bowl

Prep time: 5 minutes | Cook time: 0 minutes | Serves 8

8 medium firm and ripe pears, peeled
1/2 cup sliced cranberries
3/4 cup maple syrup
1/4 teaspoon ground ginger

1/4 teaspoon ground cinnamon
1/8 teaspoon ground cloves
Juice of 1 lemon
2 tablespoons lime juice

1. Stand pears upright in a cooker. Sprinkle with cranberries.
2. In a small bowl, combine maple syrup, ginger, cinnamon, and cloves, and spoon on top of pears.
3. Pour lemon and lime juice evenly over pears.
4. Cover and cook on low for 30 minutes

Healthy Golden Apple and Lemony Date Mix

Prep time: 5 minutes | Cook time: 30 minutes | Serves 6

6 cups cored, peeled, and thinly sliced Golden Delicious apples
2 teaspoons lemon juice
1/3 cup chopped dates
11/3 cups finely chopped almonds
1/2 cup almond flour
1/2 cup maple syrup
1/2 teaspoon ground cinnamon
1/2 teaspoon ground ginger
1/8 teaspoon ground nutmeg
1/8 teaspoon ground cloves
4 tablespoons grass-fed butter

1. Combine apples, lemon juice, and dates in a large bowl, and mix well. Transfer mixture to a cooker.
2. In a separate medium bowl, combine almonds, flour, maple syrup, cinnamon, ginger, nutmeg, and cloves.
3. Cut in grass-fed butter with two knives or a pastry blender.
4. Sprinkle nut mixture over apples and smooth down.
5. Cook on low for 30 minutes.
6. Serve warm.

Easy Cinnamon Peach Dessert

Prep time: 5 minutes | Cook time: 30 minutes | Serves 8

2 (16-ounce) packages frozen peaches, thawed and drained
3/4 cup plus 1 tablespoon maple syrup, divided
2 teaspoons ground cinnamon, divided
1/2 teaspoon ground nutmeg
3/4 cup almond flour
6 tablespoons coconut butter
1 fresh peach, cut into slices
Sprig of mint

1. Combine peaches, 3/4 cup maple syrup, 11/2 teaspoons cinnamon, and nutmeg in a large bowl. Transfer to a cooker.
2. In a separate small bowl, combine flour with remaining 1 tablespoon maple syrup and 1/2 teaspoon cinnamon.
3. Cut in coconut butter with two knives or a pastry blender and then spread mixture over peaches.

4. Cover and cook on high for 30 minutes.
5. Garnish around the cobbler with fresh peaches and put a sprig of mint leaves in the center.
6. Serve warm.

Vanilla flavoured Butter Coconut Dessert

Prep time: 5 minutes | Cook time: 30 minutes | Serves 3

3 large overripe bananas, peeled
2 tablespoons coconut butter
2 tablespoons grass-
fed butter
1/3 cup maple syrup
1 teaspoon vanilla extract

1. In a medium bowl, mash bananas with a fork or potato masher.
2. Transfer mashed bananas to a cooker.
3. Mix in coconut butter, grass-fed butter, maple syrup, and vanilla.
4. Cover and cook on low for 30 minutes.

Mom's Special Blueberry Coconut Muffins

Prep time: 5 minutes | Cook time: 30 minutes | Serves 8

4 cups fresh blueberries
1/4 cup maple syrup, if needed
11/2 teaspoons vanilla
1 tablespoon lemon juice
1 cup chopped pecans
1 cup unsweetened shredded coconut
1/3 cup coconut flour
3 tablespoons coconut oil
3 tablespoons grass-fed butter
1/8 teaspoon salt

1. Preheat oven to 400°F. Grease an 8" square glass pan with coconut oil.
2. Combine blueberries, maple syrup (if using), vanilla, and lemon juice in the pan and toss gently; set aside.
3. In a medium bowl, combine pecans, coconut, and coconut flour.
4. Add coconut oil, grass-fed butter, and salt and mix until crumbly.
5. Sprinkle over blueberries.
6. Bake for 25-30 minutes or until blueberry mixture is bubbly. Serve warm or cool.

Easy Sweetie Chocolate Coconut Drops

Prep time: 5 minutes | Cook time: 10 minutes | Makes 48 drops

21/2 cups unsweetened shredded coconut

1/2 cup chocolate
2/3 cup coconut flour

1. In large heavy saucepan, melt all but 1/2 cup chocolate over low heat, stirring frequently, until melted and smooth.
2. Remove pan from heat and stir in reserved chocolate.
3. Stir constantly until mixture is smooth again.
4. Add coconut and mix well.
5. Drop mounds of this mixture onto parchment paper.
6. Let stand until set. Store in airtight container at room temperature for up to several days.

Easy Maple Blackberry Dessert

Prep time: 5 minutes | Cook time: 0 minutes | Serves 6

2 cups blackberries
1/4 cup maple syrup

1/4 cup water

1. Place all ingredients in a cooker.
2. Cook for 30 minutes.

Homemade Maple Cherry and Apple Puree

Prep time: 5 minutes | Cook time: 30 minutes | Serves 6

5 large Golden Delicious apples, peeled, cored, and sliced

2 tablespoons water
1/4 cup maple syrup
1/2 cup cherry purée

1. Place apple slices in a cooker greased with coconut oil.
2. Add water and maple syrup and toss to coat apples.
3. Cover and cook for 30 minutes.
4. Stir in cherry purée. Serve warm or allow cooling and serving chilled.

Vegan Blueberry Plum Coconut Bake

Prep time: 5 minutes | Cook time: 30 minutes | Serves 8

8 medium plums, stones removed, sliced
2 cups blueberries
2 tablespoons maple syrup
2 tablespoons lemon juice
1 tablespoon arrowroot powder
1 cup unsweetened

coconut flakes
1 cup rolled oats
1 cup chopped pecans
2/3 cup coconut flour
1/4 teaspoon baking soda
1/2 teaspoon cream of tartar
1/4 teaspoon salt
1/3 cup coconut oil, melted

1. Preheat oven to 350°F. Grease a 9" square baking dish with coconut oil.
2. Combine plums and blueberries in prepared dish.
3. Drizzle with maple syrup, lemon juice, and arrowroot powder and toss to coat.
4. In a medium bowl, combine coconut flakes, oats, pecans, coconut flour, baking soda, cream of tartar, and salt.
5. Add coconut oil and mix until crumbly. Pat mixture on top of fruit in dish.
6. Bake for 25–30 minutes or until fruit is bubbly and topping is golden. Serve warm.

Golden Apple with Coconut Butter

Prep time: 5 minutes | Cook time: 30 minutes | Serves 8

4 medium Granny Smith apples, peeled, cored, and sliced
4 medium Golden Delicious apples, peeled, cored, and sliced

3/4 cup maple syrup
1/2 teaspoon ground cinnamon
1/2 teaspoon ground cloves
1/2 cup coconut butter

1. Place apples in a 4-quart slow cooker and toss with remaining ingredients.
2. Cover and cook for 30 minutes. Serve warm.

Easy Baked Pink Apple with Coconut Butter

Prep time: 5 minutes | Cook time: 30 minutes | Serves 6

6 large Pink Lady apples
1/2 cup unsweetened coconut flakes
1/2 cup rolled oats
2 tablespoons maple syrup
1/2 teaspoon ground cinnamon
3 tablespoons coconut butter

1. Preheat oven to 350°F.
2. Remove cores from apples, leaving 1/2" intact at the bottom. Place apples in a medium baking dish.
3. In a small bowl, mix together coconut flakes, oats, maple syrup, and cinnamon. Fill cavities with mixture.
4. Top each apple with a spoonful of coconut butter.
5. Bake for 20–30 minutes. Apples are done when they are completely soft and brown on top.

Homemade Honey Nuts Bar

Prep time: 5 minutes | Cook time: 15 minutes | Serves 8

1 tablespoon honey
4 tablespoons coconut oil
1/4 cup ground almonds
1/4 cup ground hazelnuts
1/4 cup sunflower seeds
1/4 cup cacao powder
3/4 cup unsweetened coconut flakes

1. Melt honey and coconut oil in a small saucepan over medium heat.
2. In a medium mixing bowl, combine almonds, hazelnuts, sunflower seeds, cacao powder, and coconut. Mix thoroughly.
3. Add honey mixture to bowl and mix well.
4. Pour dough into an 8"× 8" greased baking pan and refrigerate or freeze until firm, about 10 minutes.
5. Cut into eight squares and serve immediately or store in refrigerator for up to several days.

Chilled Vanilla Strawberry Ice Cream

Prep time: 5 minutes | Cook time: 30 minutes | Serves 6

2 cups coconut cream
13/4 cups frozen strawberries
3/4 cup coconut sugar
2 teaspoons vanilla
1/4 teaspoon salt

1. Combine all ingredients in a food processor or blender. Purée until smooth and creamy.
2. Transfer mixture to a large freezer-proof baking or casserole dish and place in freezer.
3. Stir mixture every 10 minutes until a smooth ice cream forms, about 30 minutes. If mixture gets too firm to stir, transfer to a blender, process until smooth, then return to freezer for up to several months.

Chilled Maple Apricot Bowl

Prep time: 5 minutes | Cook time: 30 minutes | Serves 6

2/3 cup water
2/3 cup maple syrup
2 teaspoons minced fresh ginger
5 cups chopped apricots, fresh or frozen
3 tablespoons lemon juice

1. In a small saucepan over medium-high heat, bring water, maple syrup, and ginger to a boil, and then reduce heat to low.
2. Simmer for 3–4 minutes until a syrup forms. Allow to cool.
3. Combine maple syrup mixture, apricots, and lemon juice in a food processor or blender. Purée until smooth.
4. Transfer mixture to a large freezer-proof baking or casserole dish and place in freezer.
5. Stir mixture every 10 minutes until frozen and smooth, about 30 minutes.
6. If mixture gets too firm, transfer to a blender, process until smooth, then return to freezer for up to several months.

Lemony Coconut Mango Bowl

Prep time: 5 minutes | Cook time: 0 minutes | Serves 6

3 cups chopped peeled mangoes
1/2 cup cold water
1 cup unsweetened

shredded coconut
2 tablespoons lemon juice

1. In a food processor or blender, combine mangoes and water; process until smooth.
2. Add coconut and lemon juice; process until smooth.
3. Transfer to a plastic container and freeze until solid, about 2 hours.
4. Store in freezer up to several months.

Classic Raspberry Watermelon Bowl

Prep time: 5 minutes | Cook time: 0 minutes | Serves 4

4 cups chopped watermelon
1 cup raspberries
1/4 cup maple syrup

2 tablespoons lemon juice
1/8 teaspoon salt

1. In two batches, combine watermelon, raspberries, maple syrup, lemon juice, and salt in a blender or food processor.
2. Blend or process until smooth.
3. Pour mixture into a 9" square baking dish. Freeze for 3 hours, then remove from freezer and use a fork to scrape mixture into small pieces, paying special attention to the sides of the baking dish to be sure to scrape all of the mixture.
4. Return to freezer and freeze for another hour.
5. Scrape mixture again with a fork.
6. Serve immediately, or spoon lightly into a medium bowl and freeze, covered, for up to two days.
7. Scrape with a fork into serving dish and eat immediately.

Delicious Maple Cooked Apple Wedges

Prep time: 5 minutes | Cook time: 30 minutes | Serves 4

1 teaspoon maple syrup
1 tablespoon ground cinnamon
2 tablespoons lemon

juice
2 tablespoons water
4 medium apples, peeled, cored, and cut into wedges

1. Place maple syrup, cinnamon, lemon juice, and water in a cooker.
2. Stir until maple syrup dissolves. Add apples.
3. Cook for 30 minutes. Stir before serving.

Cinnamon Bosc Pear Ice Bowl

Prep time: 5 minutes | Cook time: 30 minutes | Serves 6

1 pound Bosc pears, peeled and cored
11/4 cups water
1/4 cup maple syrup

1/2 teaspoon ground cinnamon
1 tablespoon lemon juice

1. Place pears, water, maple syrup, and cinnamon in a cooker. Cover and cook on high for 30 minutes. Stir in lemon juice.
2. Process pear and syrup mixture in a blender until smooth. Strain mixture through a sieve and discard any pulp.
3. Pour liquid into an 11" × 9" baking dish, cover tightly with plastic wrap, and transfer to freezer.
4. Stir every hour with a fork, crushing any lumps as it freezes.
5. Freeze 3–4 hours or until firm. To serve, scoop into six individual small bowls.
6. Store in a tightly sealed container in the freezer for up to several months.

Cinnamon Apple Ice Bowl

Prep time: 5 minutes | Cook time: 30 minutes | Serves 6

1 pound Golden Delicious apples, peeled, cored, and chopped
11/4 cups water
1/4 cup maple syrup
1/2 teaspoon ground cinnamon
1 tablespoon lemon juice

1. Place apples, water, maple syrup, and cinnamon in a cooker. Cover and cook on high for 30 minutes. Stir in lemon juice.
2. Process apple and syrup mixture in a blender until smooth.
3. Strain mixture through a sieve, and discard any pulp.
4. Pour liquid into an 11" × 9" baking dish, cover tightly with plastic wrap, and transfer to freezer.
5. Stir with a fork, crushing any lumps as it freezes.
6. Freeze 3–4 hours or until firm. To serve, scoop into six individual small bowls.
7. Store in a tightly sealed container in the freezer for up to several months.

Super Tasty Maple Cooked Ripe Plums

Prep time: 5 minutes | Cook time: 30 minutes | Serves 4

1/2 cup maple syrup
1 cup water
1/8 teaspoon salt
1 tablespoon fresh lemon juice
1 cinnamon stick
1 pound fresh ripe plums (about 8 small or 6 medium), pitted

1. Combine all ingredients in a cooker and cook on low for 30 minutes, or until plums are tender.
2. Serve warm, chilled, or at room temperature.

Tender Grape Nectarine and Peaches Bowl

Prep time: 5 minutes | Cook time: 25 minutes | Serves 6

4 medium peaches, pitted and cut into quarters
4 medium nectarines, pitted and cut into quarters
6 large apricots, pitted and cut in half
1 tablespoon olive oil
2 tablespoons lemon juice
1/2 teaspoon salt
1/2 teaspoon dried thyme leaves
1/8 teaspoon ground white pepper
11/2 cups red grapes

1. Preheat oven to 400°F. Place peaches, nectarines, and apricots, cut side up, in a large roasting dish.
2. Drizzle with olive oil and lemon juice.
3. Sprinkle with salt, thyme, and white pepper.
4. Roast, uncovered, for 15 minutes.
5. Add grapes to the pan and stir gently.
6. Roast for another 5–10 minutes or until fruit is tender.

Easy Tasty Rhubarb Bowl

Prep time: 5 minutes | Cook time: 30 minutes | Serves 4

1 pound strawberries, diced
1/2 pound rhubarb, diced
2 tablespoons lemon juice
1 tablespoon lemon zest

1. Place all ingredients in a cooker. Cook on low for 20 minutes.
2. Lightly mash with a potato masher.
3. Cook on high, uncovered, for 10 minutes.

CHAPTER 8: SALADS, DRESSINGS, SOUPS AND STOCKS

Ultimate Gazpacho dressed with Sunflower Seeds

Prep time: 7 minutes | Cook time: 5 minutes | Serves 2

8 very ripe plum or heirloom tomatoes
1 medium red bell pepper, seeded and coarsely chopped
1 medium cucumber, coarsely chopped
1/2 Cup extra-virgin

olive oil
1 Tablespoon balsamic or red wine vinegar
Salt
Freshly ground black pepper
Pepitas or sunflower seeds, for garnish

1. Add the tomatoes, pepper, and cucumber to a blender or food processor and pulse a few times to break down.
2. With the motor running, add the oil and process until very smooth and velvety, at least 2 minutes.
3. Add the vinegar and process briefly to combine.
4. Refrigerate the soup for at least 2 hours.
5. Serve cold with salt and pepper to taste and garnish with the seeds.

Per Serving

Calorie 376| Fats 34g| Carbs 20g| Protein 4g

Hazelnut Cardamom Salad Dressing

Prep time: 15 minute | Cook time: 0 minute | Serves 6

1/3 cup maple syrup
1/4 cup apple cider vinegar
2 tablespoons hazelnut oil
3 tablespoons olive oil

1/2 teaspoon cinnamon
1/8 teaspoon cardamom
1/8 teaspoon salt

1. In a small jar with a tight-fitting lid, combine all ingredients and shake well.
2. Use immediately, or cover and store in the refrigerator for up to one week.

Per Serving

Calorie 147| Fats 11g| Carbs 12g| Protein 0g

Creamy Broccoli Red Onion Salad

Prep time: 5 minutes | Cook time: 0 minutes | Serves 4

1/2 cup extra-virgin olive oil
2 tablespoons apple cider vinegar
1 Teaspoon Dijon mustard
¼ Teaspoon salt
¼ Teaspoon freshly

ground black pepper
4 cups broccoli florets
½ cup finely diced red onion
¼ cup raw or roasted unsalted sunflower seeds

1. In a large bowl, add the dressing ingredients and whisk until creamy.
2. Add the broccoli, onion, and sunflower seeds, tossing to coat.
3. Refrigerate for at least 1 hour, up to overnight.

Per Serving

Calorie 402| Fats 37g| Carbs 16g| Protein 7g

Easy Homemade Oregano Salad Dressing

Prep time: 15 minute | Cook time: 0 minute | Serves 8

1/3 cup apple cider vinegar
1/2 teaspoon dry mustard
1 teaspoon lemon juice
2 cloves garlic, peeled and chopped

1 teaspoon dried oregano
1/2 teaspoon salt
1/2 teaspoon ground black pepper
1/2 cup extra-virgin olive oil

1. Place all ingredients except olive oil in a blender. With the blender running on a medium setting, slowly pour in oil. Blend until smooth.
2. Serve immediately on salad or cover and store in the refrigerator for up to seven days.

Per Serving

Calorie 121| Fats 14g| Carbs 0g| Protein 0g

Boiled Asparagus Salad with Quick Pickled Red Onions

Prep time: 10 minutes | Cook time: 35 minutes | Serves 5

1 bunch asparagus, woody ends trimmed	mustard
3 Tablespoons extra-virgin olive oil	¼ Teaspoon salt
1 lemon	¼ Teaspoon freshly ground black pepper
2 tablespoons lemon juice	1 Pinch red pepper flakes (optional)
2 Teaspoon Dijon	Sunflower seeds, for garnish

1. Bring a large pot of salted water to a boil.
2. Add asparagus and boil until bright green and crisp tender, 2 minutes.
3. Drain and immediately rinse under cold running water or submerge in an ice bath until cool.
4. Transfer to the refrigerator to cool completely, 30 minutes.
5. To make the dressing, vigorously whisk together the remaining ingredients (minus the seeds) until emulsified, or shake in a closed jar.
6. To serve, divide asparagus among plates and drizzle with 2 tablespoons of the dressing.
7. Garnish with seeds for crunch or with Quick-Pickled Red Onions if you have them on hand.

Per Serving

Calorie 207 | Fats 22g| Carbs 5g| Protein 3g

Creamy Curry Dressing

Prep time: 15 minute | Cook time: 0 minute | Serves 3

3 tablespoons olive oil	powder
3 tablespoons fresh lime juice	1/2 teaspoon ground black pepper
1 teaspoon curry	1 teaspoon dried basil

1. Combine all ingredients in a small bowl and stir well.

Per Serving

Calorie 122| Fats 14g| Carbs 0g| Protein 0g

Fresh Raspberry and Dijon mustard Marinade

Prep time: 15 minute | Cook time: 0 minute | Serves 10

1/4 cup apple cider vinegar	mustard
2 tablespoons lime juice	1 tablespoon maple syrup
1/4 cup raspberry purée	3/4 cup olive oil
2 tablespoons Dijon	1 teaspoon salt
	1/2 teaspoon ground black pepper

1. Process together vinegar, lime juice, raspberry purée, mustard, and maple syrup in a food processor or blender until smooth.
2. Slowly add olive oil a few drops at a time on high speed to allow oil to emulsify. Season with salt and black pepper.

Per Serving

Calorie 155| Fats 16g| Carbs 2g| Protein 0g

Sweet & Spicy Mango Cantaloupe Salad

Prep time: 15 minute | Cook time: 15 minute | Serves 4

2 tablespoons mango juice	Hungarian paprika
1 tablespoon walnut oil	1/8 teaspoon ground red pepper
1/8 teaspoon chili powder	3 cups cubed cantaloupe
1/8 teaspoon sweet	1/2 cup peeled, diced red onion

1. Whisk mango juice, oil, chili powder, paprika, and red pepper together in a small bowl until oil is emulsified.
2. Place cantaloupe and red onion in a large bowl. Pour dressing over salad and toss well to coat.
3. Cover salad and chill in refrigerator for 15 minutes. Remove bowl from refrigerator, toss gently, and serve.

Per Serving

Calorie 83| Fats 4g| Carbs 13g| Protein 1g

Five minute Sesame Dressing

Prep time: 15 minute | Cook time: 30 minute | Serves 3

2 tablespoons olive oil
2 tablespoons sesame oil
2 tablespoons tahini
1/2 teaspoon ground black pepper
1 teaspoon dried thyme leaves

1. Combine all ingredients in a small bowl and stir well.

Per Serving

Calorie 219| Fats 23g| Carbs 2g| Protein 2g

Carrot – Bell pepper Cauliflower Salad

Prep time: 15 minute | Cook time: 20 minute | Serves 4

1 medium head cauliflower, shredded
4 tablespoons lemon juice, divided
1 tablespoon coconut oil
4 medium stalks celery, sliced
1 medium yellow bell pepper, seeded and chopped
2 medium carrots,
peeled and shredded
1/3 cup finely chopped dill pickle
1/3 cup extra-virgin olive oil
1 tablespoon maple syrup
1 tablespoon chopped fresh dill
1/4 teaspoon salt
1/8 teaspoon ground black pepper

1. Toss shredded cauliflower with 1 tablespoon lemon juice.
2. Heat coconut oil in medium skillet over medium heat.
3. Add shredded cauliflower and cook for 1–2 minutes or until crisp-tender.
4. Scrape cauliflower into a large bowl and set aside to cool for 15 minutes.
5. Stir celery, bell pepper, carrots, and dill pickle into cauliflower.
6. In a small bowl, combine olive oil, remaining 3 tablespoons lemon juice, maple syrup, dill, salt, and black pepper and mix well.
7. Pour over salad and stir to coat.
8. Cover and chill for 1–3 hours before serving.

Per Serving

Calorie 284| Fats 22g| Carbs 20g| Protein 5g

Instant Spicy Cucumber Onion Salad

Prep time: 15 minute | Cook time: 0 minute | Serves 2

2 medium cucumbers, peeled and thinly sliced
3/4 teaspoon salt
1/4 cup apple cider vinegar
1 tablespoon maple syrup
1 teaspoon sesame oil
1/4 teaspoon crushed red pepper flakes
1/2 medium onion, peeled and thinly sliced

1. In a large shallow container or on a large baking sheet, spread cucumbers in a single layer and sprinkle with salt. Allow to sit at least 10 minutes.
2. Drain excess water from cucumbers. Transfer cucumbers to a medium bowl.
3. In a small bowl, whisk together vinegar, maple syrup, oil, and red pepper flakes.
4. Pour dressing over cucumbers, add onion, and toss gently.
5. Allow to sit at least 10 minutes before serving to allow flavors to mingle.

Per Serving

Calorie 95| Fats 3g| Carbs 17g| Protein 2g

Easy Cheesy Broccoli & Raisin Salad

Prep time: 15 minute | Cook time: 0 minute | Serves 4

4 tablespoons olive oil
3/4 cup pine nuts
2 cups broccoli florets
2 tablespoons raisins
1 ounce feta cheese
Juice of 1 large lemon

1. Heat olive oil in a small skillet over medium heat and sauté pine nuts until golden brown.
2. Mix broccoli, raisins, and feta cheese in a medium bowl.
3. Add pine nuts and toss.
4. Squeeze lemon juice over salad and serve.

Per Serving

Calorie 329| Fats 31g| Carbs 13g| Protein 5g

Super Tasty Quinoa Walnut Salad

Prep time: 15 minute | Cook time: 15 minute | Serves 4

1 cup uncooked quinoa
2 cups water
1 medium head green leaf lettuce, chopped
2 tablespoons chopped fresh mint
2 large tangerines, peeled and sectioned
1/3 cup chopped walnuts
1 bulb fennel, thinly sliced
2 tablespoons olive oil
1 teaspoon salt
1/2 teaspoon ground black pepper

1. Fill medium pot with water, add quinoa and bring to a boil.
2. When water boils, reduce heat to low and cover; simmer 15 minutes.
3. Remove from heat and keep covered an additional 5 minutes; then fluff with a fork and set aside.
4. Gently toss together quinoa, lettuce, mint, tangerines, walnuts, and sliced fennel.
5. Drizzle with olive oil, season with salt and black pepper, and serve immediately.

Per Serving
Calorie 330| Fats 16g| Carbs 40g| Protein 10g

Paleo Baby Greens & Raspberries Goat Cheese Salad

Prep time: 15 minute | Cook time: 30 minute | Serves 4

4 tablespoons lime juice
4 tablespoons olive oil
1/4 teaspoon ground cumin
2 teaspoons minced jalapeño pepper
4 cups mixed baby greens
2 cups raspberries
1/4 cup peeled, thinly sliced red onion
1 ounce crumbled goat cheese

1. Place lime juice, olive oil, cumin, and jalapeño in a blender and blend until smooth.
2. In a large bowl, toss dressing with greens, berries, and onions. Top with goat cheese and serve immediately.

Per Serving
Calorie 184| Fats 15g| Carbs 11g| Protein 3g

Zucchini Carrot Squash Salad

Prep time: 15 minute | Cook time: 0 minute | Serves 6

2 medium zucchini
2 large carrots, peeled
2 medium yellow summer squash
2 tablespoons olive oil
3 tablespoons lemon juice
1 tablespoon Dijon mustard
1 tablespoon chopped fresh dill
1/2 teaspoon salt
1/8 teaspoon ground black pepper

1. Rinse vegetables and pat dry; cut off ends. Using a vegetable peeler or a mandolin, shave vegetables into thin, wide ribbons.
2. In a large bowl, combine olive oil, lemon juice, mustard, dill, salt, and black pepper and mix well.
3. Add vegetable ribbons and toss to coat.
4. Serve immediately, or cover and refrigerate for up to 24 hours before serving.

Per Serving
Calorie 89| Fats 5g| Carbs 9g| Protein 3g

Healthy Creamy Broccoli Salad

Prep time: 5 minutes | Cook time: 0 minutes | Serves 4

1/2 cup extra-virgin olive oil
2 tablespoons apple cider vinegar
1 Teaspoon Dijon mustard
¼ Teaspoon salt
¼ Teaspoon freshly
ground black pepper
4 cups broccoli florets
½ cup finely diced red onion
¼ cup raw or roasted unsalted sunflower seeds

1. In a large bowl, add the dressing ingredients and whisk until creamy.
2. Add the broccoli, onion, and sunflower seeds, tossing to coat.
3. Refrigerate for at least 1 hour, up to overnight.

Per Serving
Calorie 402| Fats 37g| Carbs 16g| Protein 7g

Cashew Papaya Nutty Fruity Salad

Prep time: 15 minute | Cook time: 0 minute | Serves 4

1/2 medium pineapple, peeled, cored, and cubed	seedless grapes
1 medium papaya, peeled and cubed	1 tablespoon maple syrup
1 medium banana, peeled and sliced	1/4 cup chopped cashews
1/2 cup halved	1/4 cup unsweetened coconut flakes

1. Combine all ingredients in a large bowl, toss, and serve.

Per Serving

Calorie 229| Fats 8g| Carbs 40g| Protein 4g

Vegetable Broth Soup with Butternut Squash

Prep time: 30 minutes | Cook time: 30 minutes | Serves 8

2 medium butternut squash	onion, chopped
Salt and pepper to taste	1 tart green apple, cored and chopped
2 tablespoons olive oil	3 cups vegetable broth
1 medium yellow	2 cups water

1. Preheat the oven to 425°F and line a rimmed baking sheet with foil.
2. Cut the squash in half and place them on the baking sheet – brush the cut sides with oil and season with salt and pepper to taste.
3. Roast for 15 to 20 minutes until very tender then set aside to cool.
4. Heat the oil in a Dutch oven over medium-high heat.
5. Add the onion, apple, salt and pepper and cook for 6 to 8 minutes until softened.
6. Stir in the squash, vegetable broth and water – season with salt and pepper to taste.
7. Bring to a boil then reduce heat and simmer for 10 to 12 minutes.
8. Remove from heat and puree the soup using an immersion blender.

Per Serving

Calorie 95| Fats 4g| Carbs 13g| Protein 3g

Milky Watermelon Salad

Prep time: 15 minute | Cook time: 0 minute | Serves 6

2 tablespoons lemon juice	1/8 teaspoon salt
2 tablespoons maple syrup	3 cups cubed cantaloupe
2 tablespoons canned full-fat coconut milk	3 cups cubed watermelon
2 tablespoons chopped fresh mint	2 cups cubed honeydew melon

1. In large serving bowl, combine lemon juice, maple syrup, coconut milk, mint, and salt and mix well.
2. Add melons and stir gently to coat.
3. Serve immediately, or cover and chill for up to 6 hours before serving.

Per Serving

Calorie 92| Fats 1g| Carbs 221g| Protein 2g

Epic Sea Lettuce with Tender Edamame Dressing

Prep time: 15 minute | Cook time: 30 minute | Serves 4

1/4 cup wakame seaweed	edamame, thawed
1/2 cup sea lettuce	1/4 cup orange juice
3 cups chopped kale	7 tablespoons sesame seeds, divided
1/2 teaspoon lemon juice	1 tablespoon kelp powder
1 cup frozen shelled	

1. Soak wakame and sea lettuce in water for 30 minutes. Rinse vegetables and discard the soak water.
2. Place kale in a large bowl and sprinkle with lemon juice.
3. Massage juice into kale until kale is wilted. Add wakame, sea lettuce, and edamame.
4. Place orange juice, 6 tablespoons sesame seeds, and kelp powder in a blender and blend until smooth.
5. Pour dressing over kelp mixture and toss to coat.
6. Top with remaining sesame seeds.

Per Serving

Calorie 184| Fats 12g| Carbs 11g| Protein 10g

Sweet & Delicious Onion Salad Dressing

Prep time: 15 minute | Cook time: 0 minute | Serves 10

1 small onion, peeled and finely chopped
2 cloves garlic, peeled and minced
1/4 cup apple cider vinegar
1 tablespoon lemon juice
2 tablespoons tomato paste
2 tablespoons

Homemade Ketchup
1 tablespoon Dijon mustard
21/2 tablespoons maple syrup
1/2 cup olive oil
1/2 teaspoon smoked paprika
1/4 teaspoon salt
1/8 teaspoon ground white pepper

1. Combine all ingredients in a food processor or blender.
2. Cover and blend until smooth.
3. Cover and refrigerate for 2–3 hours to let flavors blend.
4. Store tightly covered in the refrigerator for up to five days.

Per Serving
Calorie 120| Fats 11g| Carbs 6g| Protein 0g

Tender Vegetables Soup

Prep time: 15 minute | Cook time: 10 minute | Serves 4

1 large head cauliflower, chopped
3 large stalks celery, chopped
1 medium carrot, peeled and chopped
2 cloves garlic, peeled and minced
1 medium onion,

peeled and chopped
2 teaspoons ground cumin
1/2 teaspoon ground black pepper
1 tablespoon chopped parsley
1/4 teaspoon dill

1. In a large soup pot or Dutch oven, combine cauliflower, celery, carrot, garlic, onion, cumin, and black pepper.
2. Add water to just cover ingredients in pot. Bring to a boil over high heat.
3. Reduce heat to low. Simmer about 8 minutes or until vegetables are tender.
4. Stir in parsley and dill before serving.

Per Serving
Calorie 62| Fats 1g| Carbs 13g| Protein 4g

Carrot Papaya and Butternut Squash Salad

Prep time: 15 minute | Cook time: 15 minute | Serves 4

3 cups peeled and cubed butternut squash
2 tablespoons olive oil, divided
2 medium carrots, peeled and shredded
2 cups diced papaya

2 tablespoons shredded fresh ginger
Juice of 1 medium lime
1 tablespoon honey
1 teaspoon salt
1/2 teaspoon ground black pepper

1. Preheat oven to 425°F. Place squash on a large baking sheet and drizzle with 1 tablespoon olive oil. Roast for 15 minutes or until tender.
2. Remove from oven and cool.
3. In a large salad bowl, combine squash, carrots, and papaya. Set aside.
4. In a small bowl, stir together ginger, lime juice, honey, remaining 1 tablespoon olive oil, salt, and black pepper until well combined.
5. Toss the dressing with the squash mixture and serve.

Per Serving
Calorie 210| Fats 7g| Carbs 39g| Protein 2g

Instant Cantaloupe Blueberry Salad

Prep time: 15 minute | Cook time: 0 minute | Serves 4

11/2 cups cubed cantaloupe
1 cup cubed seedless watermelon
1 cup halved green grapes

3/4 cup blueberries
1 tablespoon minced mint leaves
1 teaspoon minced flat-leaf parsley

1. In a large salad bowl, gently toss cantaloupe, watermelon, grapes, and blueberries together.
2. Add mint and parsley to salad. Toss to combine.
3. Serve immediately or chill for up to 2 hours before serving.

Per Serving
Calorie 79| Fats 0g| Carbs 18g| Protein 3g

Garlicky Vegetable Stock

Prep time: 15 minute | Cook time: 30 minute | Serves 4

3 medium carrots, peeled and coarsely chopped
3 medium parsnips, peeled and coarsely chopped
3 large onions, peeled and quartered
3 whole medium turnips
3 medium rutabagas, quartered
3 medium bell peppers, seeded and halved
2 medium shallots, peeled
1 medium head garlic
1 medium bunch fresh thyme
1 medium bunch parsley
5 quarts water

1. Preheat oven to 425°F. Line a 9" × 13" baking pan with parchment paper. Arrange all the vegetables and herbs in the pan and roast for 15 minutes or until browned. Flip vegetables halfway through.
2. Add vegetables to a 6-quart slow cooker.
3. Add 5 quarts water and cover.
4. Cook on low for 15 minutes
5. Strain stock, discarding the solids. Freeze or refrigerate stock and use within one to two weeks.

Per Serving
Calorie 64| Fats 0g| Carbs 15g| Protein 2g

Peppery Balsamic Marinade

Prep time: 15 minute | Cook time: 0 minute | Serves 8

1/4 cup apple cider vinegar
3/4 cup olive oil
1 tablespoon Dijon mustard
1/4 teaspoon salt
1/8 teaspoon ground black pepper
1/2 teaspoon dried basil
1/2 teaspoon dried parsley

1. In a small bowl, whisk together all ingredients with a fork until well combined.

Per Serving
Calorie 182| Fats 20g| Carbs 0g| Protein 0g

Rich Garlic Thyme Mushroom Stock

Prep time: 15 minute | Cook time: 30 minute | Serves 4

1 quart water
12 ounces white mushrooms
6 parsley stems (with leaves)
1 large onion, peeled and sliced
1 large leek (white part only)
1 medium stalk celery, sliced
2 ounces dried
shiitake mushrooms
1 tablespoon minced garlic
11/2 teaspoons black peppercorns
3/4 teaspoon dried sage
3/4 teaspoon dried thyme leaves
1/2 teaspoon ground black pepper

1. Combine all ingredients except ground pepper in a 6-quart slow cooker; cover and cook on low for 30 minutes.
2. Strain, discarding solids; season with ground pepper.
3. Serve immediately, refrigerate and use within one to two weeks, or freeze up to several months.

Per Serving
Calorie 46| Fats 0g| Carbs 9g| Protein 2g

Healthy Cumin Cauliflower Soup

Prep time: 15 minute | Cook time: 30 minute | Serves 4

1 pound cauliflower florets
1 (14-ounce) can cannellini beans, drained and rinsed
21/2 cups water
1 medium onion,
peeled and minced
2 cloves garlic, peeled and minced
3 teaspoons curry powder
1/4 teaspoon cumin

1. Place all ingredients in a 4-quart slow cooker. Stir. Cook on low for 30 minutes.
2. Use an immersion blender to purée the soup or blend the soup in batches in a blender until smooth.

Per Serving
Calorie 110| Fats 1g| Carbs 20g| Protein 7g

Almond Tomato Onion Soup

Prep time: 15 minute | Cook time: 20 minute | Serves 4

4 cups chopped tomatoes	Vegetable Stock
1/2 cup peeled, chopped onion	2 tablespoons olive oil
4 whole cloves	2 tablespoons almond flour
2 cups Basic	Juice from 1 medium lime

1. In a stockpot, combine tomatoes, onion, cloves, and vegetable stock over medium-high heat. Bring to a boil, reduce heat to medium-low, and simmer for about 20 minutes.
2. Remove from heat and strain into a large bowl. Discard solids.
3. In the now-empty stockpot, combine olive oil and almond flour. Stir until mixture thickens.
4. Gradually whisk in tomato mixture and stir in lime juice.

Per Serving

Calorie 144| Fats 9g| Carbs 15g| Protein 3g

Easy Spicy Zucchini Coconut Milk Soup

Prep time: 15 minute | Cook time: 25 minute | Serves 8

4 cups sliced, peeled zucchini	1 teaspoon dried marjoram leaves
4 cups Basic Vegetable Stock	1/4 teaspoon celery seeds
4 cloves garlic, peeled and minced	1/2 cup canned full-fat coconut milk
2 tablespoons lime juice	1/4 teaspoon cayenne pepper
2 teaspoons curry powder	1 teaspoon paprika

1. Combine all ingredients except coconut milk, cayenne pepper, and paprika in a 4–6-quart slow cooker, and cook on high for 25 minutes
2. Process zucchini mixture with coconut milk in a blender until combined.
3. Season with cayenne pepper. Sprinkle with paprika and serve warm.

Per Serving

Calorie 58| Fats 3g| Carbs 8g| Protein 2g

Coriander Squash Coconut Soup

Prep time: 15 minute | Cook time: 30 minute | Serves 6

2 cups Roasted Vegetable Stock	1/4 teaspoon ground coriander
2 medium acorn squash, peeled, seeded, and cut into cubes	1/4 teaspoon ground cumin
1/2 cup peeled, chopped onion	1/2 cup canned full-fat coconut milk
1/2 teaspoon ground cinnamon	1 tablespoon lemon juice
	1 teaspoon ground black pepper

1. Combine stock, squash, onion, cinnamon, coriander, and cumin in a 4-quart slow cooker.
2. Cover and cook on high for 30 minutes.
3. Blend squash mixture, coconut milk, and lemon juice in a food processor until smooth.
4. Season with pepper before serving.

Per Serving

Calorie 117| Fats 3g| Carbs 22g| Protein 2g

Homemade Peppercorn Vegetable Stock

Prep time: 15 minute | Cook time: 30 minute | Serves 4

2 pounds yellow onions, peeled and roughly chopped	roughly chopped
1 pound carrots, peeled and roughly chopped	11/2 gallons water
	1 cup chopped parsley stems
1 pound celery,	4 sprigs fresh thyme
	2 bay leaves
	15 peppercorns

1. Place onions, carrots, celery, and water in a large stockpot over medium heat; bring to a simmer and cook, uncovered, for 25 minutes.
2. Add parsley stems, thyme, bay leaves, and peppercorns, and continue to simmer, uncovered, for 5 minutes.
3. Remove from heat and strain stock. Discard solids. Stock can be refrigerated for two to four days or frozen for up to three months.

Per Serving

Calorie 40| Fats 0g| Carbs 9g| Protein 1g

Mushroom Thyme and Celery Soup

Prep time: 15 minute | Cook time: 25 minute | Serves 6

2 tablespoons olive oil	6 cups Basic
1 medium shallot, peeled and finely minced	Vegetable Stock
	1 teaspoon dried thyme leaves
1 (8-ounce) package cremini mushrooms, sliced	1 teaspoon salt
	1/8 teaspoon ground white pepper
1 medium bunch celery, trimmed and thinly sliced	1 tablespoon lemon juice

1. In large pot, heat olive oil over medium heat. Add shallot; cook until softened, about 3 minutes.
2. Add mushrooms; cook and stir until mushrooms give up their liquid, about 8 minutes.
3. Add celery and cook for 4 minutes longer.
4. Add stock, thyme, salt, and white pepper, and bring to a simmer.
5. Cover pot, reduce heat to low, and simmer for 15–20 minutes or until soup is blended. Stir in lemon juice and serve immediately.

Per Serving

Calorie 100| Fats 5g| Carbs 13g| Protein 3g

Lemony Tarragon Salad dressing

Prep time: 15 minute | Cook time: 0 minute | Serves 8

2 tablespoons Dijon mustard	juice
	4 teaspoons chopped fresh tarragon
2 tablespoons apple cider vinegar	2/3 cup olive oil
1 tablespoon lemon	1/4 teaspoon salt

1. In a small jar with screw-on lid, combine all ingredients. Cover jar tightly and shake well.
2. Store in refrigerator for up to one week; shake before each use.

Per Serving

Calorie 163| Fats 18g| Carbs 0g| Protein 0g

Kale Pesto Almond Soup

Prep time: 15 minute | Cook time: 15 minute | Serves 6

3 tablespoons olive oil	5 cups Basic
1 medium onion, peeled and chopped	Vegetable Stock
	2/3 cup almond butter
2 cloves garlic, peeled and minced	1/3 cup unsweetened almond milk
1 medium jalapeño pepper, seeded and minced	1/2 teaspoon salt
	1/8 teaspoon ground black pepper
3 tablespoons almond flour	2/3 cup sliced almonds, toasted
1 teaspoon ground cumin	1/2 cup Kale Pesto

1. In large soup pot, heat olive oil over medium heat.
2. Add onion, garlic, and jalapeño; cook and stir for 5 minutes.
3. Add almond flour and cumin; cook for 1 minute. Then beat in stock and simmer for 2 minutes until thickened.
4. Add almond butter, almond milk, salt, and black pepper. Simmer for 10 minutes until flavors are blended.
5. In a small bowl combine almonds with Kale Pesto and mix.
6. Serve soup with this mixture for topping.

Per Serving

Calorie 396| Fats 33g| Carbs 20g| Protein 11g

Guava Strawberries & Peach Soup

Prep time: 15 minute | Cook time: 30 minute | Serves 4

2 cups cubed cantaloupe	2 tablespoons fresh lime juice
2 cups cubed peaches	1 cup sliced strawberries
11/2 cups guava nectar	

1. Combine cantaloupe, peaches, guava nectar, and lime juice in a blender or food processor and purée until smooth. Chill.
2. To serve, spoon soup into individual bowls and garnish with strawberry slices.

Per Serving

Calorie 146| Fats 1g| Carbs 36g| Protein 2g

Authentic Lemony Tomato Soup

Prep time: 15 minute | Cook time: 0 minute | Serves 6

1 (28-ounce) can chopped tomatoes
1 medium green bell pepper, seeded and chopped
3 medium tomatoes, peeled and chopped
1 large cucumber, peeled and chopped
1 small onion, peeled and chopped
2 tablespoons olive oil
1/2 teaspoon ground

black pepper
1/2 teaspoon paprika
1/4 teaspoon cayenne pepper
1 teaspoon chopped chives
2 teaspoons chopped parsley
1/2 clove garlic, peeled and minced
41/2 teaspoons lemon juice

1. Blend canned tomatoes in blender until smooth.
2. Pour into a large bowl.
3. Add remaining ingredients to bowl and stir to combine.
4. Refrigerate at least 12 hours. Serve chilled.

Per Serving
Calorie 90| Fats 5g| Carbs 11g| Protein 2g

Creamy Sweet Potato Mango Soup

Prep time: 15 minute | Cook time: 30 minute | Serves 4

3 large sweet potatoes, peeled and cubed
2 cups Roasted Vegetable Stock
1 (15-ounce) can

sliced mangoes, untrained
1/4 teaspoon ground allspice
1/2 cup canned full-fat coconut milk

1. Place all ingredients except coconut milk in a 4-quart slow cooker.
2. Cover and cook on low for 30 minutes.
3. When sweet potatoes are soft, purée soup in a blender and stir in coconut milk.

Per Serving
Calorie 230| Fats 5g| Carbs 45g| Protein 4g

Steamed Cauliflower with Roasted Butternut Squash

Prep time: 30 minutes | Cook time: 30 minutes | Serves 4

1 Tablespoon olive oil
Salt and black pepper
¼ cup red onion — chopped
1 Tablespoon green onions, chopped
1 medium cauliflower head, cut into florets
1 small butternut squash, peeled and

cut in cubes
1 Teaspoon garlic, minced
1/2 cup Vegenaise or traditional mayonnaise
2 tablespoons Dijon mustard
Salt and pepper

1. First, steam the head of cauliflower.
2. Add about 2 cups of water in a large pot and place a steamer basket in the bottom.
3. Bring the water to a boil.
4. Add the cauliflower florets into the steamer basket.
5. Cover the pot and steam until the cauliflower florets are tender 6-8 minutes. The time will depend on how tender you prefer your cauliflower florets to be.
6. Remove from the heat and also remove the lid from the pot. Let the cauliflower cool down for 5 minutes.
7. While the cauliflower florets are been steamed, roast the butternut squash.
8. Preheat oven to 400 degrees. On a baking sheet lined with parchment paper or silicone mat, place butternut squash and toss in olive oil and season with salt and black pepper. Mix well to combine.
9. Roast in the oven for 15-20 minutes
10. Place the steamed cauliflower, the roasted butternut squash and the red onions in a bowl.
11. Add all the ingredients in a small glass bowl for the dressing and whisk everything together to combine.
12. Taste to check the seasoning and pour over the salad.
13. Mix all the ingredients together until well combined and garnish it with green onions.

Per Serving
Calorie 287| Fats 22g| Carbs 13.3g| Protein 4g

Kale and Golden Beets Peppery Salad

Prep time: 30 minutes | Cook time: 10 minutes | Serves 3

6 red or golden beets
1 head garlic
½ Cup plus
2 Teaspoons extra-virgin olive oil, divided
1 bunch kale (or 6 to 8 cups baby kale)
2 tablespoons apple cider vinegar or red

wine vinegar
½ Teaspoon salt
½ Teaspoon freshly ground black pepper, or to taste
¼ cup raw sunflower seeds, pepitas, or pistachios (optional)

1. Preheat the oven to 375°F.
2. Slice the tops off the beets and wash thoroughly.
3. Wrap each beet with aluminum foil and place on a baking sheet or roasting pan.
4. Slice off the top of the garlic.
5. Place the head of garlic in the center of a small square of foil.
6. Drizzle 1 Teaspoon of the oil over the top of the garlic and fold the sides of the foil to wrap into a ball.
7. Set the wrapped garlic on one side of the pan with the beets.
8. Roast until the beets are tender when pierced with a paring knife, 45 to 60 minutes.
9. Remove from the oven, open the foil pouches, and let cool.
10. While the beets and garlic cool, tear the kale leaves off the ribs and then tear the leaves into smaller pieces.
11. Massage the leaves with 1 Teaspoon of the oil to soften and remove bitterness.
12. When cool enough to handle, peel the beets using your hands and a towel under cold running water.
13. Cut the beets into small wedges and set aside.
14. To make the dressing, squeeze the garlic cloves into a blender.
15. When the garlic is no longer steaming, add ⅓ cup oil, the vinegar, salt, and pepper, and purée until smooth.
16. To serve, toss the kale and beets with half of the dressing and divide among 4 shallow bowls.
17. Top evenly with sunflower seeds or goat cheese, if desired.
18. Season with more black pepper and enjoy.

Per Serving
Calorie 476 | Fats 28g| Carbs 51g| Protein 11g

Sweet and Toasted Pumpkin Soup

Prep time: 15 minute | Cook time: 30 minute | Serves 6

1 medium sugar pumpkin, peeled, seeded, and chopped (reserve seeds)
1/4 teaspoon salt
3 medium leeks, sliced
11/2 teaspoons minced fresh ginger
2 tablespoons olive

oil, divided
1/2 teaspoon grated lemon zest
1 teaspoon lemon juice
2 quarts Basic Vegetable Stock
1 teaspoon ground black pepper

1. Preheat oven to 375°F.
2. Clean pumpkin seeds thoroughly, place them on a baking sheet, and sprinkle with salt to taste. Roast for approximately 5–8 minutes, until light golden. Remove from oven and set aside.
3. Place chopped pumpkin in a large baking dish with leeks, ginger, and 1 tablespoon olive oil; roast for 20 minutes or until tender.
4. Transfer the cooked pumpkin mixture to a large stockpot and add zest, juice, stock, and black pepper. Bring to a boil over medium-high heat. Reduce heat to low and simmer for 10 minutes.
5. To serve, ladle into serving bowls.
6. Drizzle with remaining olive oil and sprinkle with toasted pumpkin seeds.

Per Serving
Calorie 141| Fats 5g| Carbs 23g| Protein 3g

CHAPTER 9: SIDE DISHES

Easy and Healthy Fried Cauliflower

Prep time: 10 minutes | Cook time: 10 minutes | Serves 4

1 head fresh cauliflower, greens removed, washed
1 tablespoon coconut oil or extra-virgin
olive oil
Salt, to taste
Freshly ground black pepper, to taste

1. Break the cauliflower into florets, put in a food processor, and pulse in 1-second intervals 10 to 15 times, until the cauliflower resembles rice.
2. Alternately, grate the florets using the medium-size slots of a box grater.
3. Heat the coconut oil in a large skillet over medium heat until melted.
4. Add the cauliflower, cover, and cook until softened and the odour dissipates, 5 to 8 minutes.
5. Remove the lid, season with salt and pepper, and fluff with a fork.

Three ingredients Vegetables Fruit Salad

Prep time: 15 minute | Cook time: 30 minute | Serves 4

1 large head red cabbage, sliced
2 medium onions, peeled and chopped
6 small tart apples, peeled, cored, and quartered
1 cup hot water
1 cup apple juice
2 tablespoons maple syrup
2/3 cup lime juice
1/2 teaspoon caraway seeds
3 tablespoons grass-fed butter, melted
3 tablespoons olive oil

1. Place cabbage, onions, and apples in a cooker that has been greased with coconut oil.
2. In a medium bowl whisk together water, apple juice, maple syrup, lime juice, and caraway seeds. Pour over cabbage.
3. Drizzle butter and olive oil over everything and cover cooker. Cook on high for 30 minutes. Stir well before serving.

Simple and Easy Tender Lemony Artichokes

Prep time: 15 minute | Cook time: 30 minute | Serves 4

3 large artichokes
1 cup water
1 large lemon, cut into eighths
2 tablespoons lemon juice
1 teaspoon dried oregano

1. Place artichokes stem side down in a cooker.
2. Pour water into the bottom of the slow cooker.
3. Add lemon slices, lemon juice, and oregano.
4. Cook on high for 30 minutes or until leaves are tender.

Three-Pepper Garlic Dish

Prep time: 15 minute | Cook time: 30 minute | Serves 4

1/4 cup olive oil
2 large green bell peppers
2 large yellow bell peppers
2 large red bell peppers
6 cloves garlic, peeled and minced
1 teaspoon ground black pepper

1. Preheat grill or broiler and Pour olive oil into a large bowl.
2. Dip peppers in olive oil, then place peppers on grill or a broiler pan. Reserve remaining oil.
3. Grill or broil peppers, turning frequently, until skin is blistered and beginning to blacken.
4. Place peppers in a paper bag and fold over the top of the bag.
5. Let peppers steam in the bag for 10 minutes.
6. Remove peppers from bag and peel off the blistered skin.
7. Slice peppers and return them to the bowl with olive oil, along with garlic and black pepper.
8. Serve at room temperature or store in the refrigerator for up to three days.

Tender Carrot Coconut Curry

Prep time: 3 minutes | Cook time: 15 minutes | Serves

1 pound carrots, peeled
3 tablespoons coconut oil
¼ teaspoon salt
¼ teaspoons freshly ground black pepper
1 cup full-fat coconut milk or water

1. Slice the carrots at an angle into 2½-inch pieces.
2. Heat the coconut oil in a large Dutch oven or skillet over medium heat.
3. Add the carrots and turn to coat; season with the salt and pepper.
4. Pour in the coconut milk and bring to a boil.
5. Reduce the heat to a simmer, cover, and cook until the carrots are just tender, 7 to 10 minutes.
6. Remove the lid, increase the heat, and continue to cook until the water fully evaporates, then serve.

Spicy Peppery Green Beans with Baby Peas

Prep time: 15 minute | Cook time: 15 minute | Serves 4

1 pound fresh green beans, trimmed and chopped
1 tablespoon olive oil
1 tablespoon sesame oil
1 (10-ounce) package frozen baby peas, thawed
4 cloves garlic, peeled and minced
1 teaspoon minced fresh ginger
1/2 teaspoon crushed red pepper flakes
1 teaspoon salt
1/2 teaspoon ground black pepper

1. Fill a medium saucepan with cold salted water and bring to a boil over high heat.
2. Add beans and cook until they are a vibrant green, about 3–4 minutes.
3. Drain and rinse under cold water.
4. Heat olive oil and sesame oil in a large skillet.
5. Add green beans, peas, garlic, ginger, and red pepper flakes.
6. Cook, stirring frequently, for 10 minutes until garlic is soft.
7. Season with salt and black pepper.

Pepper Roasted Squash

Prep time: 10 minutes | Cook time: 30 minutes | Serves 2

2 medium delicate squash (about 2 pounds)
1 tablespoon extra-virgin olive oil
1 tablespoon maple syrup
¼ teaspoon salt
¼ teaspoon freshly ground black pepper

1. Preheat the oven to 425°F.
2. Slice each squash lengthwise in half. Scoop out the seeds. Flip the squash, cut-side down, and slice into 1-inch pieces.
3. Place the squash on a baking sheet and toss with the olive oil and maple syrup until evenly coated.
4. Spread out the squash in a single layer so the pieces do not overlap.
5. Roast until tender and browned, flipping once halfway, 20 to 25 minutes.
6. Season with the salt and peppers.

Classic Root Vegetables Recipe

Prep time: 15 minute | Cook time: 30 minute | Serves 4

1 pound parsnips, peeled and diced
1 pound turnips, peeled and diced
2 medium onions, peeled and chopped
1 pound carrots, peeled and diced
6 dried apricots, chopped
4 pitted prunes, chopped
1 teaspoon ground turmeric
1 teaspoon ground cumin
1/2 teaspoon ground ginger
1/2 teaspoon ground cinnamon
1/4 teaspoon ground cayenne pepper
1 tablespoon dried parsley
1 tablespoon dried cilantro
14 ounces Basic Vegetable Stock

1. Add parsnips, turnips, onions, carrots, apricots, prunes, turmeric, cumin, ginger, cinnamon, cayenne pepper, parsley, and cilantro to a cooker.
2. Pour in stock. Cover and cook on low for 30 minutes or until vegetables are cooked.

Five Spiced Almonds Celery Fry

Prep time: 15 minute | Cook time: 10 minute | Serves 4

2 tablespoons olive oil
2 cloves garlic, peeled and minced
3 cups sliced celery
1/4 cup water
1 tablespoon coconut amino
1/2 teaspoon five-

spice powder
1/2 cup chopped celery leaves
1/8 teaspoon crushed red pepper flakes
1/3 cup sliced almonds, toasted

1. In a large saucepan, heat olive oil over medium heat.
2. Add garlic; cook for 1 minute.
3. Add celery; cook for 2–3 minutes or until crisp-tender.
4. Add water and coconut amino; bring to a simmer.
5. Cover pan, reduce heat, and simmer for 4 minutes.
6. Uncover pan and add five-spice powder, celery leaves, and crushed red pepper flakes; cook for 2 minutes longer.
7. Sprinkle with almonds and serve immediately.

Crispy Onion and Tender Apple Mix

Prep time: 15 minute | Cook time: 15 minute | Serves 4

1 tablespoon grass-fed butter
1 tablespoon olive oil
2 medium onions, peeled and chopped
2 cloves garlic, peeled and minced
3 medium apples, peeled, cored, and

sliced
3 tablespoons maple syrup
1 tablespoon lemon juice
1/2 teaspoon salt
1/2 teaspoon dried thyme leaves

1. In a large saucepan, melt butter and olive oil over medium heat.
2. Add onions and garlic and cook until crisp-tender, about 4 minutes.
3. Add apples and stir.
4. Drizzle with maple syrup and lemon juice, and sprinkle with salt and thyme leaves.
5. Cover and cook on low for about 7–9 minutes or until apples are tender. Serve immediately.

One Pan Mushroom with Sautéed Almonds

Prep time: 15 minute | Cook time: 10 minute | Serves 4

1 pound fresh green beans, trimmed and chopped
2 tablespoons olive oil
1/3 cup sliced almonds
3/4 cup sliced

mushrooms
1/2 medium yellow onion, peeled and chopped
1/2 teaspoon lemon juice

1. Fill a medium saucepan with cold salted water and bring to a boil over high heat.
2. Add beans and cook until they are a vibrant green, about 3–4 minutes.
3. Drain and rinse under cold water.
4. Heat olive oil in a large skillet over medium heat.
5. Sauté almonds, mushrooms, and onion for 3–4 minutes, stirring frequently.
6. Add green beans and lemon juice and heat for another 2 minutes.

Spicy Onion Collard Greens Mix

Prep time: 15 minute | Cook time: 30 minute | Serves 4

2 tablespoons olive oil
1 medium onion, peeled and diced
3 cloves garlic, peeled and minced
1 pound collard greens, chopped
3/4 cup water

1 (14-ounce) can diced tomatoes, drained
11/2 teaspoons Cajun seasoning
1/2 teaspoon hot sauce
1/4 teaspoon salt

1. In a large skillet, heat olive oil over medium heat.
2. Add onion, garlic, and collard greens and sauté for 3–5 minutes until onions are soft.
3. Add water, tomatoes, and Cajun seasoning.
4. Bring to a simmer over low heat, cover, and allow to cook for 20 minutes, or until greens are soft, stirring occasionally.
5. Remove lid, stir in hot sauce and salt, and cook, uncovered, for another 1–2 minutes, to allow excess moisture to evaporate.

Hot and Spicy Garlic Broccoli with Bell Peppers

Prep time: 15 minute | Cook time: 15 minute | Serves 4

1 medium head broccoli
2 tablespoons coconut oil
1 medium onion, peeled and chopped
1 medium red bell pepper, seeded and chopped
1 medium orange bell pepper, seeded and chopped
3 cloves garlic, peeled and sliced
3 tablespoons water
1/2 teaspoon salt
1/8 teaspoon ground black pepper

1. Cut the florets off the broccoli stems. Peel stems and cut into 1" slices.
2. In a medium saucepan, steam broccoli until crisp-tender, about 3–4 minutes. Drain and set aside.
3. In a large skillet, melt coconut oil over medium heat. Add onion and cook for 3 minutes.
4. Add bell peppers and cook for another 3 minutes, stirring occasionally. Add broccoli, garlic, water, salt, and black pepper to skillet.
5. Bring to a simmer, then cover and simmer for 3–4 minutes until everything is hot.

Roasted Apples Brussels Mix

Prep time: 15 minute | Cook time: 25 minute | Serves 4

2 cups quartered Brussels sprouts
8 cloves garlic, peeled
2 tablespoons olive oil
2 tablespoons apple cider vinegar
3/4 teaspoon salt
1/2 teaspoon ground black pepper
2 medium apples, peeled, cored, and chopped

1. Preheat oven to 425°F.
2. Arrange Brussels sprouts and garlic in a single layer on a large baking sheet.
3. Drizzle with olive oil and apple cider vinegar and season with salt and black pepper.
4. Roast for 10–12 minutes, tossing once.
5. Remove tray from oven and add apples, tossing gently to combine.
6. Roast for 10 more minutes or until apples are soft, tossing once again.

Seasonal Vegetable Mix

Prep time: 10 minutes | Cook time: 10 minutes | Serves 4

2 tablespoons extra-virgin olive oil
1 small onion, chopped
1 small eggplant, unpeeled, cut into ½-inch cubes
1 large red bell pepper, seeded and cut into ½-inch pieces
1 large zucchini, cut into ½-inch cubes
6 to 8 ripe tomatoes cut into ½-inch pieces, reserving the juices
¼ cup packed fresh basil leaves, chopped
¼ teaspoon salt
¼ teaspoons freshly ground black pepper

1. Heat the olive oil in a large, deep skillet or Dutch oven over medium heat.
2. Add the onion and eggplant and cook, stirring occasionally, until the onion is slightly browned and the eggplant is tender, about 5 minutes.
3. Add the bell pepper and zucchini and cook, stirring occasionally, until tender, about 10 minutes.
4. Stir in the tomatoes and their juices, cover, and simmer until the vegetables are tender and the ratatouille thickens, 5 minutes.
5. Remove the lid, stir in the basil, and season with the salt and pepper.
6. Serve warm or cover and chill for at least 1 hour or up to overnight to serve cold; this allows the flavors to meld.

Onion Black pepper Corn Salad

Prep time: 15 minutes | Cook time: 0 minutes | Makes 2 cup

1 large red onion, diced into ½-inch pieces
2 cups apple cider
vinegar
1 teaspoon salt
1 tablespoon whole black peppercorns

1. In a large glass jar or bowl with a lid, add the onions, vinegar, salt, and pepper. Give the mixture a quick stir.
2. Cover and refrigerate overnight. The onions will keep in the refrigerator for about 3 weeks.

Tender Tomato Asparagus with pepper

Prep time: 15 minute | Cook time: 30 minute | Serves 4

1 pound asparagus, trimmed
1 (28-ounce) can petite diced tomatoes
1/2 cup peeled, chopped onion
4 cloves garlic, peeled and minced
3/4 teaspoon dried oregano
3/4 teaspoon basil
1 teaspoon ground black pepper

1. Combine all ingredients except pepper in a smaller slow cooker and cover.
2. Cook on high for about 30 minutes or until asparagus is tender. Season with pepper.

Tender Orangey Butternut Squash

Prep time: 15 minute | Cook time: 30 minute | Serves 4

5 cups peeled, seeded, and cubed butternut squash
1/4 cup maple syrup
1 tablespoon orange zest
1/2 teaspoon ground cinnamon
1/2 teaspoon ground cloves

1. Add all ingredients to a greased (with coconut oil) cooker.
2. Cook on high for 30 minutes until squash is fork tender.

Low Sodium Turnip Salad

Prep time: 15 minute | Cook time: 30 minute | Serves 4

4 medium turnips, peeled and cubed
2 tablespoons olive oil
2 tablespoons maple syrup
1 tablespoon brown mustard
1/4 teaspoon ground black pepper

1. Place turnips in a cooker, drizzle with olive oil and toss.
2. In a small bowl, mix together remaining ingredients.
3. Drizzle over turnips and mix well.
4. Cover and cook on low for 30 minutes.

Roasted Carrot Parsnips & Sweet Potato Bowl

Prep time: 15 minute | Cook time: 30 minute | Serves 4

3 medium carrots, peeled and chopped
2 small parsnips, peeled and chopped
2 medium sweet potatoes, peeled and chopped
2 tablespoons olive oil
1 teaspoon salt
1/2 teaspoon ground black pepper
1/4 cup maple syrup
2 tablespoons Dijon mustard
1 tablespoon apple cider vinegar
1/2 teaspoon hot sauce

1. Preheat oven to 400°F.
2. On a large baking sheet, spread out carrots, parsnips, and sweet potatoes in a single layer.
3. Drizzle with olive oil and season with salt and black pepper. Roast for 40 minutes, tossing once.
4. In a small bowl, whisk together maple syrup, Dijon mustard, apple cider vinegar, and hot sauce.
5. Transfer roasted vegetables to a large bowl and toss well with maple mixture.

Quinoa and Cinnamon Butternut Squash Salad

Prep time: 15 minute | Cook time: 20 minute | Serves 4

3 cups peeled, seeded, and cubed butternut squash
1 tablespoon ground cinnamon
1 teaspoon nutmeg
2 cups water
1 cup uncooked quinoa

1. Preheat oven to 350°F.
2. Place squash in 9" × 11" baking dish. Sprinkle with cinnamon and nutmeg. Bake for 15 minutes or until tender and slightly brown.
3. Meanwhile, fill a medium pot with water, add quinoa, and bring to a boil. When water boils, reduce heat to low and cover; simmer 10 minutes.
4. Remove from heat and keep covered an additional 5 minutes; then fluff with a fork and set aside.

Maple based Walnut and Beets with Goat Cheese

Prep time: 15 minute | Cook time: 30 minute | Serves 4

11/2 pounds beets	walnuts
2 cups hot water	3 tablespoons lemon juice
1/4 cup peeled, finely chopped red onion	1 tablespoon coconut oil
2 tablespoons maple syrup	1 ounce crumbled goat cheese
2 cloves garlic, peeled and minced	1 teaspoon ground black pepper
4 tablespoons chopped toasted	

1. Combine beets and water in a 4–6-quart slow cooker. Cover and cook on high for about 15 minutes or until beets are tender.
2. Drain and peel beets and cut into 3/4" cubes. Combine cubed beets and remaining ingredients, except goat cheese and black pepper, in the cooker.
3. Cover and cook on high for 15 minutes.
4. Top with goat cheese and season with black pepper before serving.

Warm Chipotle Sweet Potatoes Mash

Prep time: 15 minute | Cook time: 30 minute | Serves 4

3 pounds sweet potatoes, peeled and cubed	11/4 teaspoons chipotle powder
11/2 tablespoons ghee	Juice from 1/2 large lime

1. In a large saucepan fitted with a steamer insert, heat 1" water over medium-high heat.
2. Place sweet potatoes in steamer and steam until soft, approximately 5–8 minutes. Transfer to a large bowl.
3. In a small saucepan, heat ghee and whisk in chipotle powder and lime juice.
4. Pour mixture over sweet potatoes and mash with fork or potato masher.

Fresh Vegan Coconut Jicama with White Pepper

Prep time: 15 minute | Cook time: 15 minute | Serves 4

1 large jicama	2 shallots, minced
1 tablespoon lemon juice	1/2 teaspoon salt
2 tablespoons coconut oil	1/8 teaspoon ground white pepper

1. Peel jicama and grate on a box grater or in the food processor.
2. Sprinkle with lemon juice and mix.
3. In a large skillet, melt coconut oil over medium heat.
4. Add shallots; cook and stir until tender, about 4 minutes.
5. Add grated jicama to the skillet; cook and stir until jicama releases some of its water and the water evaporates, about 5–6 minutes.
6. Taste jicama to see if it's tender.
7. If not, cook another 1–2 minutes. Then sprinkle with salt and white pepper and serve.

Garlicky Coconut Cabbage Curry

Prep time: 15 minute | Cook time: 15 minute | Serves 4

3 tablespoons coconut oil	3 cups chopped red cabbage
1 medium onion, peeled and chopped	1/4 cup water
3 cloves garlic, peeled and minced	1 tablespoon coconut amino
4 cups chopped green cabbage	1 teaspoon salt
	1/8 teaspoon ground black pepper

1. In a large skillet, heat coconut oil over medium heat.
2. Add onion and garlic; cook and stir until crisp-tender, about 4 minutes.
3. Add cabbages to the skillet and cook and stir for 4 minutes.
4. Add water, coconut amino, salt, and black pepper and bring to a simmer.
5. Cover and cook for 5–7 minutes longer until cabbage is tender.

Lemony Shredded Cabbage Salad

Prep time: 15 minute | Cook time: 0 minute | Serves 4

1 teaspoon celery seed
11/2 cups lime juice
11/2 teaspoons mustard seed
1 teaspoon turmeric
1 teaspoon lemon juice

8 cups shredded cabbage
2 medium green bell peppers, seeded and finely chopped
1 large onion, peeled and finely chopped

1. In a small saucepan over high heat, bring celery seed, lime juice, mustard seed, turmeric, and lemon juice to a boil.
2. Place cabbage, bell peppers, and onion in a 2-quart or smaller baking dish with a cover.
3. Pour boiling liquid over vegetables. Cover and let stand for 2 hours. Serve at room temperature or chilled. This salad will keep crisp for three to four weeks in the refrigerator.

One pan Roasted vegetables with jalapeño peppers

Prep time: 15 minute | Cook time: 30 minute | Serves 4

1/4 cup olive oil
3 tablespoons apple cider vinegar
1 tablespoon minced garlic
1 pound asparagus stem ends trimmed
1 pound mixed summer squashes, thinly sliced

1 pound mini sweet peppers, stemmed and sliced in half lengthwise
2 medium jalapeño peppers, seeded and chopped
1 teaspoon seasoning salt

1. Preheat oven to 400°F.
2. In a small bowl, mix together olive oil, vinegar, and garlic and set aside.
3. Place all vegetables in a large roasting pan and toss.
4. Pour olive oil mixture over top, lifting and gently mixing the vegetables so they are all coated with oil. Sprinkle with seasoning salt.
5. Roast uncovered for about 25 minutes or until vegetables begin to darken; stir occasionally. Serve hot.

Steamed Buttery Squash

Prep time: 15 minute | Cook time: 30 minute | Serves 4

1/4 cup maple syrup
1 teaspoon ground cinnamon
1 teaspoon ground nutmeg
2 small acorn squash,

halved and seeded
3/4 cup raisins
4 tablespoons grass-fed butter
1/2 cup water

1. In a small bowl, combine maple syrup, cinnamon, and nutmeg.
2. Spoon maple syrup mixture into the squash halves. Sprinkle with raisins.
3. Top each half with 1 tablespoon butter.
4. Wrap each squash half individually in aluminum foil and seal tightly. Pour water into a cooker.
5. Place wrapped squash, cut side up, in the slow cooker.
6. Cover and cook on high for 30 minutes or until squash is tender.
7. Open the foil packets carefully to allow steam to escape.

Garlic roasted Rabe and Kale

Prep time: 15 minute | Cook time: 30 minute | Serves 4

1 pound broccoli rabe, trimmed and cut into 2" pieces
1 pound kale, trimmed and cut into 4" pieces
2 tablespoons olive oil
1 medium onion,

peeled and chopped
3 cloves garlic, peeled and minced
2 tablespoons lemon juice
1 teaspoon salt
1/8 teaspoon ground white pepper

1. In a medium saucepan, steam broccoli rabe and kale for about 3 minutes. Drain and set aside.
2. In a large skillet, heat olive oil over medium heat.
3. Add onion and garlic; cook and stir until tender, about 5 minutes.
4. Add steamed broccoli rabe and kale to skillet; cook and stir for 3 minutes.
5. Add lemon juice, salt, and white pepper and cook for another 2–3 minutes until tender. Serve immediately.

Lemony Garlic Broccoli with Hazelnuts

Prep time: 15 minute | Cook time: 30 minute | Serves 4

2 pounds broccoli florets, washed and trimmed
12 cloves garlic, peeled
1/2 teaspoon ground
black pepper
1 cup large raw hazelnuts
2 tablespoons olive oil
Juice from 2 medium lemons

1. Place broccoli in a cooker and add garlic, pepper, hazelnuts, olive oil, and lemon juice and toss.
2. Cover and cook on high for 30 minutes
3. Serve and enjoy!

Green Beans Shallot Stir Fry

Prep time: 15 minute | Cook time: 30 minute | Serves 4

11/2 pounds fresh green beans, trimmed
3 tablespoons olive oil
3 large shallots, peeled and cut into thin wedges
6 cloves garlic, peeled
and sliced
1 tablespoon grated lemon zest
1/2 teaspoon ground black pepper
1/2 cup water

1. Place green beans in a greased (with coconut oil) cooker.
2. Add remaining ingredients over the top of the beans.
3. Cook on high for 30 minutes.
4. Serve and enjoy!

Cashew and Peppery Asparagus fry

Prep time: 15 minute | Cook time: 15 minute | Serves 4

2 tablespoons olive oil
2 tablespoons sesame oil
1 teaspoon minced fresh gingerroot
1 pound asparagus
ends trimmed and cut into 2" pieces
1 teaspoon crushed red pepper flakes
1/2 cup chopped cashews

1. Heat olive oil and sesame oil in a wok or large skillet over low heat.

2. Add ginger and stir-fry until slightly brown, about 5 minutes.
3. 2 Add asparagus and red pepper flakes, and stir-fry for 5 minutes.
4. Add cashews. Cook, stirring frequently, for about 5 minutes or until asparagus is tender.

Asian Sesame Apple Salad

Prep time: 15 minute | Cook time: 0 minute | Serves 4

2 cups packaged coleslaw mix
1 large unpeeled tart apple, cored and chopped
1/2 cup chopped celery
1/2 cup chopped green pepper
1/4 cup flaxseed oil
2 tablespoons lemon juice
1 teaspoon sesame seeds

1. In a medium bowl combine coleslaw mix, apple, celery, and green pepper.
2. In a small bowl, whisk together remaining ingredients.
3. Pour over coleslaw and toss to coat.

Vanilla Coconut Tender Squash & Walnuts

Prep time: 15 minute | Cook time: 30 minute | Serves 4

1 (2-pound) butternut squash, peeled, seeded, and cut into 1" cubes
1/2 cup water
1/2 cup maple syrup
1 cup chopped
walnuts
1 teaspoon cinnamon
4 tablespoons coconut butter
2 teaspoons grated fresh ginger
1 teaspoon vanilla

1. Grease a 4-quart slow cooker with olive oil.
2. Add squash and water to a cooker.
3. In a small bowl mix together maple syrup, walnuts, cinnamon, coconut butter, ginger, and vanilla.
4. Drizzle maple syrup mixture evenly over butternut squash.
5. Cook on high for 30 minutes, or until squash is fork tender.

Greens with Lemon wedges

Prep time: 5 minutes | Cook time: 10 minutes | Serves 2

1 large bunch (1 pound) Swiss or rainbow chard
1 large lemon
2 tablespoons extra-virgin olive oil

½ medium red onion, minced
¼ teaspoon salt
¼ teaspoons freshly ground black pepper

1. Leaves from 1 small bunch fresh herbs (parsley, cilantro, basil, or dill), minced (optional)
2. Rinse and lightly pat dry the chard (a little water helps them steam faster).
3. Slice the stems into ½-inch pieces and set aside. Tear the leafy greens into 3-inch pieces and set aside.
4. Using a zester or the fine side of a box grater, grate the lemon and set the zest aside. Cut the lemon into wedges and set aside.
5. Heat the olive oil in a large skillet or Dutch oven over medium heat.
6. When it is hot, add onion and chard stems and cook, stirring occasionally, until soft and translucent, 2 to 4 minutes.
7. Add the greens, cover, and steam until just wilted, about 1 minute. Remove the lid, add the reserved lemon zest, salt, pepper, and herbs (if using).
8. Toss to combine.
9. Serve the greens with the lemon wedges for squeezing just before enjoying.

Homemade Portabella Mushroom Green Stir Fry

Prep time: 5 minutes | Cook time: 15 minutes | Serves 2

10 ounces cremini or baby portabella mushrooms
2 tablespoons extra-virgin olive oil
¼ teaspoon salt
¼ teaspoons freshly

ground black pepper
4 cups baby greens (spinach, kale, or a mix)
1 tablespoon chopped fresh rosemary

1. Clean any dirt off of the mushrooms with a paper towel. Cut the mushrooms into ½-inch-thick slices.
2. Heat the olive oil in a large skillet over medium-high heat.
3. When it is hot, add the mushrooms in a single layer and cook, not stirring or flipping, until browned on one side, about 2 minutes.
4. Flip the mushrooms and cook until browned on the other side, about 2 minutes.
5. Reduce the heat to medium and continue to cook until the mushrooms have released their juices and are tender, another 5 to 8 minutes.
6. Season with the salt and pepper.
7. Add the baby greens, cover, and cook until just wilted, 30 to 60 seconds. Stir in the rosemary and serve.

Chickpea Carrots Mix with Yogurt Gravy

Prep time: 15 minutes | Cook time: 30 minutes | Serves 6

4 sun-dried tomatoes, chopped
½ teaspoon mustard seeds
¼ teaspoon cardamom seeds
1 teaspoon ghee (clarified butter), or as needed
2 teaspoons onion, chopped
1 teaspoon sliced ginger
1 clove garlic, chopped
1 teaspoon garam masala

1 teaspoon turmeric
½ teaspoon ground cinnamon
½ teaspoon ground cloves
1 (15 ounce) can chickpeas, drained
2 small carrots, sliced
1 Chile pepper, chopped
½ cup whole-milk yogurt, at room temperature
½ cup vegetable broth, or as needed (Optional)

1. Place sun-dried tomatoes in a bowl and cover with boiling water. Let soak until softened, about 10 minutes. Drain.
2. Crush mustard seeds and cardamom seeds using a mortar and pestle. Heat ghee in a skillet over medium heat; add crushed spices, onion, ginger, garlic, garam masala, turmeric, cinnamon, and cloves.
3. Fry until mixture is light brown in color, 3 to 5 minutes.
4. Add drained sun-dried tomatoes, chickpeas, carrots, and chile pepper; cook until softened as desired, about 25 minutes.
5. Stir in yogurt. Add broth to thin curry if necessary

Coconut Glazed Carrots

Prep time: 15 minute | Cook time: 30 minute | Serves 4

1 tablespoon coconut oil	1 teaspoon coconut amino
2 tablespoons maple syrup	1 pound carrots, peeled and chopped

1. Preheat oven to 400°F. In large ovenproof saucepan, combine coconut oil and maple syrup and heat on stovetop until melted.
2. Add coconut amino and carrots; cook and stir for 2 minutes.
3. Place the pan in the oven and roast for 15–20 minutes, turning once, or until carrots are tender and glazed. Serve immediately.

Vegan Carrots and Peas Bowl

Prep time: 15 minute | Cook time: 10 minute | Serves 4

1 cup water	peeled and julienned
2 tablespoons lemon juice	1 (10-ounce) package frozen baby peas, thawed
2 tablespoons lime juice	1 tablespoon extra-virgin olive oil
1 pound carrots,	

1. In a large saucepan over medium-high heat, combine water, lemon juice, lime juice, and carrots.
2. Cover and cook until carrots are tender, about 10 minutes. Remove from heat and cool.
3. In a medium bowl, combine carrots, peas and olive oil. Stir to coat.

Sweet Paprika Fry with Chopped Dill

Prep time: 20 minutes | Cook time: 20 minutes | Serves 2

2 large sweet potatoes (¾ pound total), peeled	¼ teaspoons freshly ground black pepper
1 tablespoon extra-virgin olive oil or melted coconut oil	½ teaspoon paprika (regular or smoked)
½ teaspoon salt	3 tablespoons chopped fresh dill (optional)

1. Preheat the oven to 425°F. Line a baking sheet with aluminum foil or parchment paper.
2. Slice the sweet potatoes lengthwise in half and then into ¼-by-¼-inch matchsticks, adding them to a large bowl of cold water to soak for a few minutes while prepping
3. Drain and dry thoroughly with paper towels.
4. Place the potatoes on the prepared baking sheet.
5. Toss with the oil and spread out in a single layer so the fries are not overlapping or touching.
6. Turn all the pieces to point in the same direction.
7. Bake for 15 minutes, remove from the oven, and flip the fries using a flat metal spatula.
8. Make sure the fries are not overlapping or touching and are facing the same direction.
9. Return to the oven and bake until the fries are browned and cooked through, another 15 minutes.
10. Turn off the oven, prop open the door, and allow the fries to cool and crisp up for 10 minutes.
11. Remove from the oven and season with the salt, pepper, and paprika (if using). Toss to coat, sprinkle with the dill (if using), and enjoy.

Orange & Tomato based Fennel

Prep time: 15 minute | Cook time: 30 minute | Serves 4

3 small fennel bulbs, halved
1 (13-ounce) can chopped tomatoes
Rind and juice from 1

small orange
2 tablespoons maple syrup
1/2 teaspoon ground black pepper

1. Place fennel in a 4–6-quart slow cooker.
2. In a large mixing bowl, combine remaining ingredients.
3. Pour mixture over fennel.
4. Cover and cook on high for 30 minutes.

Scrambled Pepper Egg

Prep time: 5 minutes | Cook time: 10 minutes | Serves 2

¼ cup vegetable oil
1 teaspoon ground turmeric
1 teaspoon ground coriander
Salt to taste

½ cup finely chopped onion
3 green Chile peppers, sliced
2 large eggs

1. Heat oil in a skillet over medium heat; add turmeric, coriander, and salt.
2. Cook and stir onion and green Chile peppers in the seasoned oil until onion is slightly tender, about 5 minutes.
3. Crack eggs into the skillet and season with salt
4. Cook and stir until eggs are set and scrambled, about 5 minutes.

Green Beans Dry Fry with Rosemary

Prep time: 15 minute | Cook time: 30 minute | Serves 4

1 pound green beans
1 tablespoon minced rosemary
1 teaspoon minced

thyme
2 tablespoons lemon juice
2 tablespoons water

1. Place all ingredients in a cooker.
2. Stir to distribute spices evenly.
3. Cook for 30 minutes or until green beans are tender.
4. Stir before serving.

Tomato & Onion Egg Stir Fry

Prep time: 15 minutes | Cook time: 10 minutes | Serves 3

2 tablespoons avocado oil, or as needed
6 eggs, beaten

4 ripe tomatoes, sliced into wedges
2 green onions, thinly sliced

1. Heat 1 tablespoon avocado oil in a wok or skillet over medium heat.
2. Cook and stir eggs in the hot oil until mostly cooked through, about 1 minute.
3. Transfer eggs to a plate.
4. Pour remaining 1 tablespoon avocado oil into wok
5. Cook and stir tomatoes until liquid has mostly evaporated, about 2 minutes.
6. Return eggs to wok and add green onions
7. Stir until eggs are fully cooked, about 5 minutes.

Easy Tasty Veggie mix

Prep time: 15 minute | Cook time: 30 minute | Serves 4

1 pound plum tomatoes, chopped
1 medium eggplant, cut into 1/2" pieces
2 medium zucchini, cut into 1/2" pieces
3 medium stalks celery, sliced
1 large onion, peeled and finely chopped
1/2 cup chopped

fresh parsley
1 teaspoon lemon juice
2 tablespoons lime juice
1 tablespoon maple syrup
1/4 cup raisins
1/4 cup tomato paste
1/4 teaspoon ground black pepper

1. Combine all ingredients in a cooker.
2. Cover and cook on low for 30 minutes.

Five Spiced Beef Stew with Potato and Zucchini

Prep time: 15 minutes | Cook time: 30 minutes | Serves 8

½ pound beef for stew, such as beef chuck roast, cut into 1-inch chunks
3 tablespoons olive oil
2 (3 inch) pieces fresh ginger root, peeled and diced
3 cloves garlic, minced
2 onions, peeled and diced
2 celery ribs, chopped
2 tablespoons curry powder, or to taste
2 teaspoons coriander powder

1 teaspoon Asian five-spice powder
1 teaspoon ground turmeric
2 carrots, peeled and sliced
Parsnips, peeled and sliced
2 potatoes, peeled and cubed
1 zucchini, sliced
2 apples - peeled, cored and chopped
1 cup raisins
1 cup cashews
½ cup water

1. Preheat oven to 350 degrees F (175 degrees C). Line a roasting pan with aluminum foil.
2. Meanwhile, heat the olive oil in a deep pot over medium-high heat.
3. Stir in the ginger, garlic, onions, and celery, and cook until vegetables soften, about 5 minutes.
4. Mix in the curry powder, coriander powder, five-spice powder, and turmeric, and toss to evenly coat the onion mixture.
5. Cook about 5 minutes more, and stir in the carrots, parsnips, potatoes, zucchini, and apples.
6. Stir in the beef with its cooking liquid, raisins, and cashews, and toss to evenly blend the spices.
7. Pour the beef and vegetable mixture into the prepared roasting pan. Drizzle 1/2 cup water over the mixture. Cover the pan with aluminum foil.
8. Bake in preheated oven until heated through, about 20 minutes

Spicy Beef and Tomato Coconut Curry

Prep time: 15 minutes | Cook time: 30 minutes | Serves 6

2 tablespoons ghee (clarified butter)
2 cloves garlic, crushed
1 large onion, finely sliced
2 Serrano peppers, thinly sliced
2 whole cloves, bruised
1 teaspoon garam masala
1 teaspoon ground coriander
½ teaspoon Chile

powder
1 teaspoon turmeric
1 ½ teaspoons ground cumin
1 ½ pounds beef tenderloin, cubed
1 teaspoon salt
1 cup chopped tomatoes
⅔ Cup coconut milk
1 (10 ounce) bag spinach
1 teaspoon lemon juice

1. Heat the ghee in a large saucepan over medium heat.
2. Stir in the garlic and onion, and cook until softened, about 5 minutes.
3. Add the Serrano, and continue to cook for another 1 minute.
4. Season with the cloves, garam masala, and coriander, Chile powder, turmeric, and cumin, cook for 2 to 3 more minutes to release the flavor.
5. Stir in the beef and salt, cook for 1 minute more.
6. Add the tomatoes, coconut milk, and spinach.
7. Bring to a simmer, then cover, and cook for 10 minutes, stirring occasionally.
8. Uncover, then stir in the lemon juice, and cook for 2 more minutes, stirring frequently, until the sauce has thickened.

Cashew Prawns with Tender Vegetables

Prep time: 15 minutes | Cook time: 20 minutes | Serves 8

2 ¼ pounds peeled and deveined medium shrimp
¼ teaspoon turmeric powder
¼ teaspoon ground red pepper
3 tablespoons cashews
5 whole cardamom pods, broken
2 (3 inch) cinnamon sticks
1 teaspoon whole black peppercorns
4 teaspoons sunflower

oil
½ red onion, diced
½ teaspoon garlic paste
¾ teaspoon ginger paste
salt to taste
½ teaspoon garam masala
1 large bay leaf
½ cup diced roma tomatoes
2 green bell peppers, seeded and diced
1 (14 ounce) can coconut milk

1. Season the shrimp with turmeric powder and Chile powder, and set aside.
2. Toast the cashews, cardamom, cinnamon, and peppercorns in a skillet over medium heat until toasted and fragrant, about 7 minutes; remove from the skillet and set aside
3. Heat the sunflower oil in a large skillet over medium-high heat.
4. Add the onion, garlic, and ginger; cook and stir until the onion has softened and begun to lose its red color, about 5 minutes.
5. Stir in the shrimp and toasted spice mixture along with the salt, garam masala, bay leaf, tomatoes, and green pepper.
6. Cook and stir until half of the shrimp has begun to turn pink, then pour in the coconut milk, cover, and bring to a simmer.
7. Cover, and reduce heat to medium-low.
8. Simmer until the shrimp are opaque and the vegetables are tender, about 5 minutes.

Very Spicy Carrot and Butternut Squash Curry

Prep time: 20 minutes | Cook time: 30 minutes | Serves 4

1 cup dry chickpeas (garbanzo beans)
2 tablespoons vegetable oil
2 onions, chopped
4 cloves garlic, minced
6 pods green cardamom
2 dried red Chile peppers, stemmed and seeded
2 teaspoons coriander seeds
2 teaspoons ground

turmeric
1 teaspoon black mustard seeds
1 tablespoon tomato paste, or more to taste
1 large butternut squash, peeled and cut into 1-inch cubes
3 carrots, chopped
1 ½ cups water, or as needed
½ bunch fresh cilantro, chopped

1. Place chickpeas in a large bowl and cover with cold water. Let soak, 8 hours to overnight.
2. Drain and rinse chickpeas under running cold water.
3. Place in a large pot, cover with several inches of water, and bring to a boil.
4. Reduce heat and simmer until chickpeas are soft, 20 to 25 minutes. Drain.
5. When chickpeas are halfway done, heat oil in a large pot and cook onions until soft and translucent, about 5 minutes.
6. Stir in garlic and cook until fragrant, about 30 seconds.
7. Add cardamom pods, Chile peppers, coriander seeds, turmeric, and mustard seeds and toast for 1 minute. Mix in tomato paste
8. Stir butternut squash and carrots into the pot.
9. Add enough water to cover vegetables halfway. Simmer over low heat, partially covered, until all the vegetables are soft.
10. Mix in cooked chickpeas shortly before serving and heat until warm. Serve sprinkled with cilantro.

CHAPTER 10: SAUCES AND SPREADS

Hazelnut Garlic Pesto

Prep time: 5 minute | Cook time: 5 minute | Makes 2 cups

2 cups packed chopped fresh kale
1 cup fresh basil leaves
1/2 cup toasted chopped hazelnuts
1 tablespoon lemon juice
1 clove garlic, peeled
and minced
1/2 teaspoon salt
1/8 teaspoon ground black pepper
1/3 cup olive oil
2 tablespoons hazelnut oil
1/4 cup water

1. Bring 2 cups water to a boil in a medium saucepan.
2. Place kale in a steamer basket or insert and put it in the pan. Cover.
3. Steam kale for 2–3 minutes or until slightly softened. Remove to a colander to drain. Press in kitchen towel to remove excess water.
4. Combine kale, basil, hazelnuts, lemon juice, garlic, salt, and black pepper in a food processor. Process until finely chopped.
5. With motor running, add olive oil and hazelnut oil gradually through the feed tube.
6. Add water as needed for desired consistency and Store, covered, in the refrigerator for up to a week or freeze for longer storage.

Sweet Orange Sauce Recipe

Prep time: 5 minute | Cook time: 30 minute | Serves 5

1/2 cup freshly squeezed orange juice
1/2 cup water
1/2 teaspoon orange zest
1/2 teaspoon maple syrup

1. Place all ingredients in a cooker.
2. Cook on high for 30 minutes.
3. Stir before serving.

Fresh Zucchini Thyme Sauce

Prep time: 10 minute | Cook time: 25 minute | Serves 4

1/2 medium onion, chopped 2 cloves garlic, pressed
1 to 2 zucchini, chunked 1/2 cup water
Three 8-ounce cans tomato sauce
1 teaspoon dried basil
1 teaspoon dried thyme
1 teaspoon dried oregano
2 to 4 drops Tabasco or 1/2 teaspoon crushed red pepper flakes

1. Sauté the onion, garlic, and zucchini in the water for about 5 minutes.
2. Add the remaining ingredients and cook, uncovered, over low heat for 15 to 20 minutes.

Tomato Onion Eggplant Pickle

Prep time: 5 minute | Cook time: 10 minute | Serves 6

1 large eggplant, pierced all over with fork
2 tablespoons extra-virgin olive oil
1/2 cup finely chopped tomato
1/4 cup peeled, finely chopped onion
1/4 cup almond
yogurt
3 cloves garlic, peeled and minced
1/2 teaspoon dried oregano leaves
2 tablespoons lemon juice
1 teaspoon ground black pepper

1. Place eggplant in a cooker, cover, and cook on low until tender, Cool to room temperature.
2. Cut eggplant in half lengthwise and remove eggplant pulp (including seeds) from peel with a spoon.
3. Mash eggplant pulp and mix with olive oil, tomato, onion, almond yogurt, garlic, and oregano.
4. Season with lemon juice and black pepper before serving.

Easy Spicy Tomato Spinach Sauce

Prep time: 5 minute | Cook time: 10 minute | Serves 8

1 (28-ounce) can crushed tomatoes, with liquid
1 (10-ounce) package frozen chopped spinach, thawed and drained
22/3 (6-ounce) cans tomato paste
1 (4.5-ounce) can sliced mushrooms, drained
1 medium onion, peeled and chopped

5 cloves garlic, peeled and minced
2 bay leaves
1/3 cup grated carrot
1/4 cup olive oil
21/2 tablespoons crushed red pepper flakes
2 tablespoons lemon juice
2 tablespoons dried oregano
2 tablespoons dried basil

1. In a cooker, combine all ingredients, cover, and cook on high for 30 minutes.
2. Serve.

Coconut Mint Cucumber Salad

Prep time: 5 minute | Cook time: 30 minute | Serves 4

1 (5-ounce) can full-fat coconut milk
1 medium cucumber, peeled and seeded
1/2 teaspoon salt
1/3 cup minced red onion
1 clove garlic, peeled and minced

2 tablespoons lemon juice
1 tablespoon chopped fresh mint
1/2 teaspoon ground cumin
1/8 teaspoon ground white pepper

1. Refrigerate the can of coconut milk for at least 8 hours. Spoon off the solids from the top; reserve the thin liquid for another use.
2. Slice cucumber thinly and sprinkle with salt.
3. Place in colander and place in the sink; let stand for 30 minutes. Rinse cucumber, drain, and pat dry with paper towels.
4. In a medium bowl, combine coconut milk solids, cucumber, red onion, garlic, and lemon juice and mix well. Stir in mint, cumin, and white pepper.
5. Cover and chill for 1 hour before serving.

Basil Pistachio Pesto

Prep time: 5 minute | Cook time: 0 minute | Makes 3 cups

1 (10-ounce) package frozen chopped spinach
11/2 cups shelled pistachios

1 cup fresh basil leaves
2/3 cup olive oil
1 teaspoon salt
1/4 cup water

1. In a blender or food processor, combine spinach, pistachios, and basil and blend until finely chopped.
2. With motor running, slowly add olive oil through the feed tube until mixture is smooth and thick.
3. Add salt. Add enough water for desired consistency.
4. Refrigerate, covered, for up to three days, or freeze for up to several months.

Super Smooth Coconut Cashew Spread

Prep time: 5 minute | Cook time: 0 minute | Serves 8

2 cups roasted cashews
11/2 teaspoons maple syrup

1/4 teaspoon salt
3 tablespoons coconut oil

1. Process cashews, maple syrup, and salt in a food processor on high speed until cashews form a thick paste.
2. Slowly add coconut oil until mixture is smooth and creamy, scraping down sides and adding a little more oil as needed.

Lemony Raspberry Sauce

Prep time: 5 minute | Cook time: 10 minute | Serves 16

12 ounces fresh raspberries
1 teaspoon lemon

juice
2 tablespoons maple syrup

1. Place all ingredients in a cooker.
2. Mash gently with a potato masher.
3. Cook on for 30 minutes uncovered.
4. Stir before serving.

Garlic Onion Tomatillo Sauce

Prep time: 5 minute | Cook time: 30 minute | Serves 4

1 teaspoon olive oil
2 cloves garlic, peeled and minced
1 medium onion, peeled and sliced
7 large tomatillos,

husked and diced
2 small jalapeño peppers, seeded and minced
1/2 cup water

1. Heat olive oil in a medium non-stick skillet over medium heat.
2. Sauté garlic, onion, tomatillos, and jalapeño peppers for 5–10 minutes, until softened.
3. Place mixture in a cooker.
4. Add water and stir. Cook for 25 minutes.

Homemade Tomato Cilantro Sauce

Prep time: 5 minute | Cook time: 10 minute | Serves 6

3 cloves garlic, peeled and minced
1 large onion, peeled and minced
1 (28-ounce) can crushed tomatoes
1 (14.5-ounce) can diced tomatoes

3 chipotle peppers in adobo, minced
1 teaspoon dried oregano
1 tablespoon minced fresh cilantro
1/2 teaspoon ground black pepper

1. Place all ingredients in a cooker. Cook for 30 minutes.
2. Stir before serving.

Sweet and Spicy Mango Sauce

Prep time: 5 minute | Cook time: 30 minute | Serves 20

1/4 cup apple cider vinegar
21/2 cups cubed mango

2 chipotle peppers in adobo, puréed
1 teaspoon maple syrup

1. Place all ingredients in a cooker. Stir.
2. Cook for 30 minutes.
3. Mash sauce with a potato masher.
4. Store in an airtight container for up to two weeks in the refrigerator.

Garlic Basil Habanero Sauce

Prep time: 5 minute | Cook time: 0 minute | Serves 6

2 cups chopped fresh basil leaves
3 medium habanero peppers, seeded and chopped

2 cloves garlic, chopped
1/4 cup lime juice
3 tablespoons olive oil

Combine all ingredients in a food processor and pulse to coarsely blend.

Sweet Three- Berry Sauce

Prep time: 5 minute | Cook time: 30 minute | Serves 12

1 cup raspberries
1 cup blackberries
1 cup golden

raspberries
1/2 cup water
1/2 teaspoon honey

1. Place all ingredients in a cooker. Lightly mash berries with the back of a spoon.
2. Cover and cook on low for 25 minutes, then uncover and cook on high for 5 minutes.

Spicy Eggplant Tahini Spread

Prep time: 5 minute | Cook time: 20 minute | Serves 8

2 medium eggplants, peeled and roughly chopped
2 tablespoons olive oil
1/4 cup tahini
2 cloves garlic, peeled and chopped
2 tablespoons lime

juice
1/2 teaspoon ground black pepper
1/2 teaspoon cumin
1 large avocado, pitted, peeled, and cubed

1. Preheat oven to 425°F.
2. In a large bowl, toss eggplant with olive oil. Place eggplant in a large roasting pan.
3. Roast, stirring occasionally, until eggplant is soft, about 15–20 minutes.
4. Remove eggplant from roasting pan and place in the bowl of a food processor.
5. Add remaining ingredients and pulse until slightly chunky.

Authentic Italian Parsley Tomato Sauce

Prep time: 5 minute | Cook time: 10 minute | Serves 8

1 tablespoon olive oil
1 large onion, peeled and diced
2 cloves garlic, peeled and minced
1 tablespoon minced fresh basil
1 tablespoon minced fresh Italian parsley
2/3 cup canned full-fat coconut milk
1 medium stalk celery, diced
1 (14.5-ounce) can whole tomatoes in purée
1 (28-ounce) can crushed tomatoes

1. Heat olive oil in a medium non-stick skillet over medium heat. Sauté onion and garlic for 5–10 minutes until soft.
2. Add onion and garlic to a cooker.
3. Add herbs, milk, celery, and tomatoes.
4. Stir to distribute spices. Cook for 25 minutes.

Cilantro Mango Onion Sauce

Prep time: 5 minute | Cook time: 0 minute | Serves 8

3 medium mangoes, peeled, pitted, and diced
1 small red onion, peeled and diced
1/2 cup chopped
fresh cilantro
1 teaspoon lime juice
1/2 teaspoon lime zest
1/2 teaspoon ground black pepper

1. Combine all ingredients in a medium bowl and stir gently to combine.
2. Serve at room temperature or refrigerate for 4 hours before serving.

Ginger Garlic Serrano Sauce

Prep time: 5 minute | Cook time: 0 minute | Serves 6

1 cup tightly packed mint leaves
2 medium Serrano chilies, seeded and chopped
4 cloves garlic, peeled
1 (1") piece fresh gingerroot, peeled and chopped
1/4 cup lime juice
2 tablespoons olive oil

1. Combine all ingredients in a food processor and pulse to coarsely blend.

Homemade Cinnamon Apple Sauce

Prep time: 5 minute | Cook time: 0 minute | Serves 4

2 cups ice water
1 tablespoon lemon juice
3 large Granny Smith apples, cored and diced
1 medium shallot, peeled and thinly
sliced
3 sprigs fresh mint, chopped
1 tablespoon lemon zest
1/4 cup golden raisins
1/2 teaspoon ground cinnamon

1. Combine water and lemon juice in a large mixing bowl.
2. Add apples and soak for 5 minutes.
3. Drain apples and mix them with remaining ingredients in a medium bowl.

Maple Fig Jam

Prep time: 5 minute | Cook time: 30 minute | Serves 25

2 pounds fresh figs
2 tablespoons minced fresh ginger
2 tablespoons lime
juice
1/2 cup water
3/4 cup maple syrup

1. Place all ingredients in a 2-quart slow cooker. Stir. Cook for 20 minutes.
2. Remove lid and cook an additional 10 minutes or until mixture has thickened.
3. Pour into airtight containers and refrigerate for up to six weeks.

Chilled Apple Berry Jam

Prep time: 5 minute | Cook time: 30 minute | Serves 80

2 pounds cooking apples, peeled, cored, and chopped
3 cups maple syrup
13/4 cups
blackberries
2 tablespoons lemon juice
1 medium lemon rind, grated

1. Place all ingredients in a cooker, cover, and cook on high 30 minutes, stirring periodically.
2. Pour jam into warmed canning jars and allow cooling.
3. Cover and store in refrigerator for up to two months.

Garlic Lemony Mint Pesto

Prep time: 5 minute | Cook time: 0 minute | Makes 2

2 cups packed fresh mint leaves	nuts
1 clove garlic, peeled	1/4 teaspoon salt
2 tablespoons lemon juice	1/3 cup extra-virgin olive oil
1/3 cup toasted pine	2–3 tablespoons water

1. In a blender or food processor, chop mint with garlic until finely chopped.
2. Add lemon juice, pine nuts, and salt and process again until finely chopped.
3. With the machine running, add olive oil and water until a sauce forms. You may need to add more water for desired consistency.
4. Store covered in the refrigerator for up to three days; freeze for longer storage for up to several months.

Homemade Medjool Date Syrup

Prep time: 5 minute | Cook time: 0 minute | Makes 3 cups

2 cups pitted Medjool dates	powder
½ teaspoon stevia	1½ to 2 cups water

1. Place all ingredients in a blender and purée until smooth and creamy.
2. Add water as needed to get the mixture to blend. Store refrigerated for up to one week.

Cilantro & Jalapeño Pepper Dip Cream

Prep time: 5 minute | Cook time: 0 minute | Makes 1 cup

1 cup Low-Fat Mayonnaise	chopped
2 jalapeño peppers, seeded and finely	4 tablespoons chopped fresh cilantro
	Zest of 2 limes

1. Combine everything in a blender and purée until smooth and creamy.
2. Store refrigerated in an airtight container for up to seven days.

Spicy Parsley Cilantro Sauce

Prep time: 5 minute | Cook time: 0 minute | Makes 2 cups

11/2 cups packed flat-leaf parsley	vinegar
1/3 cup fresh cilantro	2 tablespoons lemon juice
1 medium shallot, peeled and chopped	2/3 cup olive oil
3 cloves garlic, peeled and chopped	1/2 teaspoon salt
1/4 cup apple cider	1/8 teaspoon ground black pepper

1. Combine parsley, cilantro, shallot, and garlic in a food processor and process until finely chopped. You can chop all these ingredients by hand if you'd like.
2. Transfer to a medium bowl and add vinegar, lemon juice, olive oil, salt, and black pepper; stir with a whisk until combined.
3. Refrigerate until serving time.

Five minute Garlic Tahini Cashew Sauce

Prep time: 5 minute | Cook time: 5 minute | Serves 6

1/2 cup raw cashews	1 teaspoon minced garlic
11/4 cups water	1/2 teaspoon salt
2 tablespoons lemon juice	1/4 cup nutritional yeast
2 tablespoons tahini	2 tablespoons olive oil
1/4 cup peeled, diced onion	

1. In a blender, process cashews and water until completely smooth and creamy, about 90 seconds.
2. Add remaining ingredients except olive oil and purée until smooth.
3. Slowly add oil until mixture is thick and oil is completely blended in.
4. Heat in a medium saucepan over low heat for 4–5 minutes, stirring frequently.

Vanilla flavoured Hazelnut Avocado Jam

Prep time: 5 minute | Cook time: 5 minute | Serves 16

2 cups chopped hazelnuts	3/4 cup maple syrup
1/2 cup unsweetened cocoa powder	1/2 teaspoon vanilla
	4 tablespoons avocado oil

1. Process hazelnuts in a food processor until very finely ground, about 3–4 minutes.
2. Add cocoa powder, maple syrup, and vanilla, and process to combine.
3. Add oil a little bit at a time until mixture is soft and creamy.

Spicy Apple Pears Jam

Prep time: 5 minute | Cook time: 10 minute | Serves24

4 medium Wine sap apples, peeled, cored, and sliced	1/2 cup maple syrup
	1/4 teaspoon ginger
4 medium Bartlett pears, peeled, cored, and sliced	1/4 teaspoon cinnamon
	1/4 teaspoon nutmeg
1 cup water	1/4 teaspoon allspice

1. Place all ingredients in a cooker. Cook on low for 15 minutes.
2. Uncover and cook on low for an additional 15 minutes or until thick and most of the liquid has evaporated.
3. Allow to cool completely, and then pour into a food processor and purée.
4. Pour into medium clean glass jars. Refrigerate for up to six weeks.

Easy Spicy Smith Apple Spread

Prep time: 5 minute | Cook time: 30 minute | Serves 12

8 large Granny Smith apples, peeled, cored, and quartered	2 teaspoons ground cinnamon
	1/2 teaspoon allspice
1/2 cup unsweetened apple juice	1/2 teaspoon ground cloves
3/4 cup maple syrup	

1. Place apples and juice in a 2-quart slow cooker.

2. Cover and cook on high for 20 minutes.
3. Use an immersion blender to purée apples.
4. Stir in maple syrup, cinnamon, allspice, and cloves.
5. Reduce the temperature of the slow cooker to low.
6. Cook uncovered for 10 minutes or until apple butter is thick and dark.
7. Store in the refrigerator for several weeks or freeze for up to one year.

Magic Cauliflower Leek Sauce

Prep time: 5 minute | Cook time: 15 minute | Makes 2 cups

2 large leeks, thinly sliced	nutmeg
	2 cups Cauliflower Purée
1½ teaspoon thyme, minced	Sea salt and black pepper to taste
Pinch of ground	

1. In a large saucepan, sauté the leeks over medium heat for 7 to 8 minutes.
2. Add water 1 to 2 tablespoons at a time to keep the leeks from sticking.
3. Add the thyme and nutmeg and cook for 1 minute.
4. Add the cauliflower purée and cook over medium-low heat for 5 minutes.
5. Season with salt and pepper.

Homemade Garlic Dip Cream

Prep time: 5 minute | Cook time: 0 minute | Makes 2 Cups

1½ cups Cauliflower Purée	½ teaspoon paprika
½ teaspoon ground mustard	½ teaspoon prepared horseradish
¼ cup red wine vinegar	½ teaspoon vegan Worcestershire sauce
¼ cup tomato purée	½ cup Best Date Syrup Ever
1 clove garlic, minced	

1. Combine all ingredients in a food processor and purée until smooth and creamy.
2. Store refrigerated in an airtight container for up to seven days.

Grandma's Garlic Onion Dip Cream

Prep time: 5 minute | Cook time: 0 minute | Makes 2 cup

2 tablespoons red wine vinegar	onion
2 teaspoons Dijon mustard	1 teaspoon sea salt
2 cloves garlic, minced	1½ cups Cauliflower Purée or 1 12-ounce package firm silken tofu
1 teaspoon granulated	

1. Combine all ingredients in a food processor and purée until smooth and creamy.
2. Refrigerate.

Protein rich Garlic Edamame Dip

Prep time: 10 minute | Cook time: 0 minute | Makes 3 cups

1 pound frozen shelled edamame, thawed	cloves)
⅓ Cup tahini	2 tablespoons lemon juice (about 1 small lemon)
2 tablespoons grated fresh ginger	1 teaspoon salt
3 teaspoons minced garlic (about 3	1 tablespoon sesame oil (optional)

1. In a food processor or high-speed blender, purée the edamame, tahini, ginger, garlic, lemon juice, and salt until smooth.
2. With the motor running, slowly drizzle in the sesame oil (if using) until creamy.
3. Transfer to a storage container and seal the lid.

Hot and Spicy Onion Ground Cumin Sauce

Prep time: 5 minute | Cook time: 15 minute | Makes 3 cups

1 small yellow onion, minced	cumin
2 cloves garlic, minced	½ teaspoon oregano
1½ tablespoons ancho chili powder	3 cups Cauliflower Purée
2 teaspoons ground	Sea salt and black pepper to taste

1. Sauté the onion over medium heat for 10 minutes.

2. Add water 1 to 2 tablespoons at a time to keep the onion from sticking.
3. Add the garlic, chili powder, cumin, and oregano, and cook for another minute.
4. Add the cauliflower purée and cook for 2 to 4 minutes until the sauce is hot. Season with salt and pepper.

Quick Ginger-Garlic Miso Dressing

Prep time: 5 minute | Cook time: 30 minute | Makes 1 ¾ cups

1 cup Cauliflower Purée	peeled
⅔ cup brown rice vinegar	2 tablespoons minced fresh ginger
¼ cup mellow white miso	2 tablespoons brown rice syrup
4 large cloves garlic,	½ teaspoon cayenne pepper

1. Combine all ingredients in a food processor and purée until smooth and creamy.
2. Store refrigerated in an airtight container for up to seven days.

Quick & Fresh Thyme Tomato Sauce

Prep time: 5 minute | Cook time: 30 minute | Makes 14 cups

2 medium carrots, peeled and diced	paste
2 stalks celery, diced	1½ cups chopped fresh basil
6 cloves garlic, minced	2 teaspoons thyme, minced
12 large ripe tomatoes, chopped	2 teaspoons oregano, minced
2 tablespoons tomato	1 bay leaf

1. Sea salt and black pepper to taste
2. Sauté the onion, carrots, and celery over medium heat for 10 to 12 minutes.
3. Add water 1 to 2 tablespoons at a time to keep the vegetables from sticking.
4. Add the garlic and cook for 2 minutes.
5. Add the remaining ingredients and bring to a boil.
6. Decrease the heat to low and cook the sauce, partially covered, for 1 hour.

Spicy Vegan Paprika Garlic Cashew Cream

Prep time: 5 minute | Cook time: 0 minute | Makes 1 ½ Cups

1 cup raw cashews
2½ cups water, divided
2 tablespoons lemon juice (about 1 small lemon)
½ teaspoon salt
½ teaspoon unseasoned rice

vinegar or apple cider vinegar
2 teaspoons minced garlic (about 2 cloves)
1 teaspoon smoked paprika (optional)
1 tablespoon extra-virgin olive oil

1. In a small bowl, soak the raw cashews in 2 cups of water for 1 hour. Rinse and drain.
2. Transfer the cashews to a blender, and add the lemon juice, salt, vinegar, garlic, and paprika.
3. Blend at high speed, and slowly drizzle the olive oil into the mixture. If needed, slowly drizzle in the remaining ½ cup of water until you reach a thick, creamy consistency.
4. Transfer the cream into a glass jar. Close the lid tightly.

Barley Miso Mushroom Sauce

Prep time: 15 minute | Cook time: 30 minute | Makes 1 Quarts

13/4 cups vegetable broth or water
4 tablespoons barley miso (red or traditional)
1 onion, chopped
2 cups sliced mushrooms (about 1/2 pound)

Dash freshly ground pepper
2 to 3 teaspoons dried sage (to taste)
2 teaspoons dried thyme
4 tablespoons arrowroot, dissolved in 1/4 cup water

1. Bring the broth or water to a boil. Spoon the miso into the boiling liquid and stir to dissolve.
2. Add the onion, mushrooms, sage, and thyme. Simmer for 15 to 20 minutes, stirring occasionally.
3. Add the dissolved arrowroot to the mixture.
4. Stir until thickened, about 5 minutes.
5. Add a dash of fresh pepper and more miso if a stronger gravy taste is desired

Creamy Leek Mushroom Sage Sauce

Prep time: 10 minute | Cook time: 25 minute | Makes 2 cups

1/4 pound mushrooms (8 large), sliced
1 leek, washed and sliced
2 cups water
1 tablespoon soy sauce
Freshly ground white pepper

2 tablespoons cornstarch
1 teaspoon parsley flakes
1/4 teaspoon dried oregano
1/4 teaspoon dried sage
1/8 teaspoon paprika

1. Sauté the mushrooms and leek in 1/2 cup of the water for 5 minutes.
2. Add an additional 1 cup of water and all the seasonings.
3. Cook over low heat for 15 minutes.
4. Mix the cornstarch in the remaining 1/2 cup cold water.
5. Slowly add to the sauce while stirring. Cook, stirring, until thickened and clear.

Golden Carrot Orange Honey Sauce

Prep time: 10 minute | Cook time: 10 minute | Makes 1 ½ cups

3 tablespoons whole-wheat pastry flour
1/4 teaspoon salt (optional)
1/2 cup honey
2/3 cup boiling water
1/3 cup brandy (or
1 teaspoon brandy

extract)
1/4 cup minced carrot
2 tablespoons fresh-squeezed orange juice
2 tablespoons fresh lemon juice
Dash ground nutmeg

1. In small saucepan, combine the flour and salt. Dissolve the honey in the boiling water and add the brandy. (If extract is used, add it last and use 1/3 cup more water.)
2. Add the hot liquid mixture slowly to the flour mixture. Cook over medium heat for 5 minutes, or until thick and clear, stirring constantly.
3. Add the carrot, orange and lemon juices, and the nutmeg.
4. Simmer for 5 minutes longer

Authentic Green Chili Tomato Sauce

Prep time: 10 minute | Cook time: 30 minute | Makes 3 Quarts 2

31/2 cups water
Four 16-ounce cans whole tomatoes, chopped
Three 15-ounce cans tomato sauce
Four 7-ounce cans

chopped green chillies
2 tablespoons diced jalapeño pepper
6 cloves garlic (or 2 tablespoons garlic powder)

1. Place all of the ingredients in a large pot and cook for 30 minutes or as long as possible.
2. Add garlic powder to taste

Rich Garlic Soy Sauce

Prep time: 10 minute | Cook time: 10 minute | Serves 2

6 to 8 cloves garlic, thinly sliced
1 onion, sliced
One 8.45-ounce package low-fat plain soy milk

1 heaping tablespoon corn starch
1 heaping tablespoon brewer's yeast Garlic powder to taste (optional)

1. Sauté the garlic and onion in a small amount of water for 3 to 5 minutes.
2. In another pot, mix the soy milk, corn starch, and yeast.
3. Add the garlic, onion, and any water remaining in the sauté pan.
4. Bring to a boil and cook, stirring constantly, until thickened
5. Serve

Classic Pepper Sauce

Prep time: 10 minute | Cook time: 20 minute | Makes 1 cup

2 large red bell peppers, chopped
1 small onion, chopped
2 cloves garlic, minced
1/8 teaspoon white pepper

1/4 cup water
11/2 teaspoons white-wine vinegar
1/8 teaspoon crushed red pepper flakes
Dash or two Tabasco
1/2 to 1 tablespoon horseradish (optional)

1. Place the bell peppers, onion, and garlic in a saucepan with the water.

2. Cover and cook over low heat until the peppers are very soft, about 15 minutes.
3. Transfer to a food processor or blender and process until smooth. Return to the saucepan.
4. Add the remaining ingredients.
5. Cook over low heat for 5 minutes, stirring occasionally, to allow the flavors to blend

Creamy Garlic Cilantro Butter Dip

Prep time: 5 minute | Cook time: 30 minute | Makes 1 ½ Cups

4 bunches fresh cilantro
3 cloves garlic, peeled
3 to 4 tablespoons

fresh lemon juice
2 tablespoons honey
1 to 2 tablespoons natural peanut butter

1. Wash the cilantro well and remove any yellowed leaves and tough stems. Place in a food processor with the garlic.
2. Process until finely chopped. Combine the lemon juice, honey, and peanut butter in a bowl.
3. Combine the two mixtures and mix well.

Super Simple Marinara Bell Pepper Sauce

Prep time: 20 minute | Cook time: 30 minute | Serves 6

1 cup diced green bell pepper
1 cup diced onion
1 cup shredded carrot
1 cup shredded celery
1 cup sliced mushrooms
3 cloves garlic, minced
1 cup water
15- to 16-ounce can whole tomatoes, chopped, with liquid
One 28-ounce can crushed tomatoes or

tomato puree
1/4 cup nonalcoholic red wine
1 tablespoon parsley flakes
1 small bay leaf
3/4 teaspoon dried basil
3/4 teaspoon dried oregano
1/2 teaspoon dried thyme
1/4 teaspoon dried tarragon

1. Place the vegetables and garlic in a large pot with the water. Cook, stirring, until slightly tender, about 10 minutes.
2. Add the remaining ingredients and cook, uncovered, for 35 minutes. Remove the bay leaf before serving.

All-purpose Spicy Ketchup

Prep time: 5 minute | Cook time: 10 minute | Serves 10

1 (15-ounce) can no-salt-added tomato sauce
2 teaspoons water
1/2 teaspoon onion powder
3/4 cup maple syrup
1/3 cup lime juice
1/4 teaspoon ground cinnamon
1/8 teaspoon ground cloves
1/8 teaspoon ground allspice
1/8 teaspoon nutmeg
1/8 teaspoon ground black pepper
2/3 teaspoon sweet paprika

1. Add all ingredients to a 21/2-quart slow cooker.
2. Cover and cook for 30 minutes or until ketchup reaches desired consistency, stirring occasionally.
3. Turn off the slow cooker or remove the insert from the slow cooker. Allow mixture to cool, then put in a covered container
4. Store in the refrigerator for up to a month.

Magic Garlic Onion Artichoke Sauce

Prep time: 5 minute | Cook time: 30 minute | Serves 4

1 teaspoon olive oil
8 ounces frozen artichoke hearts, defrosted
3 cloves garlic, peeled and minced
1 medium onion, peeled and minced
2 tablespoons capers
1 (28-ounce) can crushed tomatoes

1. Heat olive oil in a large non-stick skillet over medium heat.
2. Sauté artichoke hearts, garlic, and onion for about 2-5 minutes until onions are translucent and most of the liquid has evaporated.
3. Put mixture into a cooker.
4. Stir in capers and crushed tomatoes.
5. Cook on high for 25 minutes.

Chilled Tahini Beet Smoothie

Prep time: 5 minute | Cook time: 0 minute | Serves 8

4 medium beets, scrubbed, cooked, and cubed
1/4 cup raw tahini
paste
1/4 cup lemon juice
1 small clove garlic, peeled and pressed

1. Place all ingredients in a food processor and pulse until smooth.
2. Chill and serve.

Super Tasty and Creamy Shallot Mushrooms

Prep time: 5 minute | Cook time: 30 minute | Serves 8

1 cup hot water
2 shallots, minced
8 ounces cremini mushrooms (about 3-3½ cups), sliced
4 tablespoons arrowroot powder whisked together with
¼ cup cold water
2½ cups vegetable stock or Basic Soup Stock
6 tablespoons dry sherry
Sea salt and black pepper to taste

1. Place the dried porcini mushrooms in a medium bowl and pour the hot water over them. Let stand for about 20 minutes.
2. Strain the mushrooms and reserve the liquid. Coarsely chop the mushrooms.
3. Sauté the shallots, porcini mushrooms, and cremini mushrooms over medium-high heat for 7 to 8 minutes.
4. Add water 1 to 2 tablespoons at a time as needed to keep the vegetables from sticking.
5. Add the arrowroot mixture, vegetable stock, ½ cup of the reserved porcini mushroom soaking liquid, and sherry, and bring the gravy to a boil.
6. Cook until thickened and remove from the heat. Season with salt and pepper.
7. Serve hot.

Scallions and Oyster Mushroom Sauce

Prep time: 20 minute | Cook time: 15 minute | Serves 6

4 cups water
3 ounces dried shiitake or oyster mushrooms
1 medium onion, chopped
1 bunch scallions, chopped
2 cloves garlic,

minced
11/2 tablespoons grated fresh ginger
1/3 cup soy sauce
1/4 cup sherry or rice vinegar
1/3 cup corn starch, mixed with 1/2 cup cold water

1. Boil 2 cups of the water and pour over the dried mushrooms in a bowl.
2. Soak for 15 minutes while you are chopping the vegetables.
3. Remove the mushrooms from the water and squeeze to remove excess water.
4. Strain the water and reserve 1 cup. Set aside.
5. Cut the tough stems off the mushrooms and discard.
6. Chop the mushrooms into bite-sized pieces. Set aside.
7. Put the 1 cup of reserved mushroom liquid into a saucepan. Add the chopped onion. Cook, stirring occasionally, until the onion softens, 2 to 3 minutes.
8. Add the scallions, garlic, ginger, soy sauce, sherry or rice vinegar, and the chopped mushrooms.
9. Mix well and add the remaining 2 cups of water. Heat to boiling, stirring occasionally.
10. Add the corn starch mixture and cook, stirring continually, until thickened and clear.

Hot and Spicy Yellow Pepper-Potato Puree

Prep time: 15 minute | Cook time: 30 minute | Serves 6

4 medium yellow bell peppers
2 medium potatoes
1 cup water
2 tablespoons white wine
1 tablespoon fresh

lemon juice
11/2 teaspoons soy sauce
1 teaspoon onion powder
1/4 teaspoon freshly ground white pepper

1. Clean and chop the peppers and peel and chop the potatoes. Place in a saucepan with the water.
2. Cover and cook over low heat for 30 minutes.
3. Remove from the heat. Pour into a blender or food processor. Blend until smooth.
4. Return to the saucepan and add the remaining ingredients.
5. Heat through to allow the flavors to blend.

Creamy Almond Spread

Prep time: 5 minute | Cook time: 0 minute | Serves 6

2 cups almonds   2 teaspoons olive oil

1. Place almonds in a food processor and turn on.
2. Add olive oil as needed, depending on creaminess desired.

CHAPTER 11: MEAT & CHICKEN RECIPES

Grass fed Beef /Ground chicken Chilly

Prep time: 30 minutes | Cook time: 15 minutes | Serves 2

2 red, yellow, orange, or green bell peppers
3 Tablespoons extra-virgin olive oil, divided
454 g ground chicken or ground grass-fed beef
1 Tablespoon ground cumin
1 Tablespoon chilli powder
1½ Teaspoons ground cinnamon
¼ Teaspoon salt
Teaspoon freshly

ground black pepper
Pinch cayenne pepper (optional)
1 small yellow or sweet onion, diced
2 cloves garlic, minced
6 plum tomatoes, diced, juices reserved
1 cup pitted or pimento-stuffed green olives, quartered
½ cup chopped fresh cilantro

1. Preheat the oven to 400°F.
2. Slice the peppers in half, keeping the stem intact, and remove seeds. Lightly coat with 1 Tablespoon olive oil and place on an aluminum foil–lined baking sheet, cut-side up.
3. In a medium bowl, mix the meat with the cumin, chili powder, cinnamon, salt, black pepper, and cayenne (if using).
4. Heat 1 Tablespoon of the oil in a large skillet over medium heat.
5. Add the meat and cook until lightly browned but not cooked through, about 2 minutes. Transfer to a bowl using a slotted spoon.
6. In the same skillet, heat the remaining 1 Tablespoon oil. Add the onion and cook until soft and translucent, stirring a few times, about 2 minutes. Add the garlic and cook until fragrant, about 30 seconds.
7. Stir in the tomatoes and their juices, olives, and cilantro. Spoon the mixture into the bell pepper halves.
8. Bake until the peppers are tender and any excess tomato juices have evaporated, 10 to 15 minutes. Remove from the oven; allow cooling slightly, and serving.

Per Serving
Calorie 768| Fats 49g| Carbs 29g| Protein 51g

Healthy Chicken Lettuce Paleo Salad

Prep time: 30 minutes | Cook time: 10 minutes | Serves 3

340 g skinless, boneless chicken breast halves
3 (7 inch) corn tortillas
3 cups shredded lettuce
1/4 cup and 2 tablespoons chopped fresh cilantro
2-1/4 Teaspoons lime juice
1 Tablespoon and 1-1/2 Teaspoons chilli powder
3/4 Teaspoon ground

cumin
3/4 Teaspoon ground coriander
1-1/4 Teaspoons brown sugar
1/8 Teaspoon cayenne pepper
2-1/4 Teaspoons olive oil
3/4 avocado - peeled, pitted, and sliced (optional)
3/4 lime, cut into wedges (optional)
3 Tablespoons sour cream (optional)

1. Preheat an outdoor grill for medium-high heat and lightly oil the grate.
2. In a bowl, mix black beans, salsa, 1/2 cup cilantro, and lime juice and set aside.
3. Stir chili powder, cumin, coriander, brown sugar, cayenne pepper, and olive oil in a bowl until smooth; rub mixture over chicken breasts.
4. Cook chicken breasts on a preheated grill until no longer pink in the center and the juices run clear, 10 to 12 minutes per side. An instant-read thermometer inserted into the center should read at least 165 degrees F (74 degrees C).
5. Place tortillas on the grill, while Chicken is cooking and grill until lightly brown on both sides, 3 to 5 minutes.
6. Transfer chicken to a cutting board and slice into long thin strips. Divide chicken strips over tortillas and top with bean mixture, lettuce, and remaining 1/2 cup cilantro.
7. Serve with avocado, lime wedges, and sour cream.

Per Serving
Calorie 470| Fats 18.7g| Carbs 44g| Protein 35.2g

Caramelized Apple Pork Chops with onions

Prep time: 30 minutes | Cook time: 15 minutes | Serves 2

Brined Pork
1½ cups water
½ cup apple cider vinegar
2 tablespoons salt, plus more for seasoning
1 Teaspoon freshly ground black pepper (or ½ Tablespoon peppercorns)
1 Teaspoon maple syrup
2 (2-inch-thick) bone-in pastured pork

chops
1 medium red apple
1 Teaspoon lemon juice
2 tablespoons unsalted grass-fed butter
1 Tablespoon olive oil
1 medium yellow onion, diced
2 cloves garlic, minced
2 tablespoons chopped fresh parsley (optional)

1. In a large shallow bowl, combine the water, vinegar, salt, pepper, and maple syrup and microwave on high until the salt dissolves, about 1 minute.
2. Add the pork, submerging it in the brine. Cover and refrigerate for at least an hour and up to overnight.
3. Place a baking sheet or broiler pan in the oven and set the broiler to high.
4. Remove the chops from the brine, shaking off any excess and patting dry.
5. Season each side evenly with salt and pepper and set aside to dry out further while you prepare the relish.
6. For the relish, dice the apple and toss with the lemon juice. Heat the butter and oil in a medium skillet over medium heat.
7. Add the onion and cook, stirring occasionally, until it starts to caramelize, 7 to 10 minutes. Add the garlic and cook until fragrant, about 30 seconds.
8. Reduce the heat to low, add the apple, stir to coat with the mixture, cover the pan, and cook until just warmed, 1 to 2 minutes.
9. Remove from the heat, stir in the parsley (if using), and set aside.
10. Transfer the pork chops to a baking sheet or broiler pan and broil until slightly pink in the center, about 3 minutes per side, reserving juices from the pan. Let rest for 3 minutes.
11. To serve, divide the chops between two plates. Pour any juice from the pan over the chops, top evenly with the apple-onion relish, and serve.

Per Serving
Calorie 444| Fats 28g| Carbs 25g| Protein 25g

One Pan Pork Lion with Brussels

Prep time: 30 minutes | Cook time: 10 minutes | Serves 4

454 g pork tenderloin
1 Teaspoon salt
1 Teaspoon freshly ground black pepper
1 Teaspoon paprika (regular or smoked, optional)
454 g Brussels sprouts, trimmed and halved

1 medium yellow or sweet onion, cut into ½-inch wedges
2 tablespoons extra-virgin olive oil
1 Teaspoon maple syrup
1 Tablespoon fresh rosemary, minced

1. Preheat the oven to 425°F. Line a baking sheet with aluminum foil or parchment paper.
2. Place the pork in the center of the prepared baking sheet and pat dry.
3. Mix the salt, pepper, and paprika (if using) together in a small bowl. Rub it all over the pork.
4. In a medium bowl, toss the Brussels sprouts and onion with the oil, maple syrup, and rosemary. Spoon the mixture around the pork.
5. Roast the pork and Brussels sprouts until the pork is brown outside and slightly pink inside (internal temperature should be 145°F).
6. Remove from the oven and let rest for 3 minutes.
7. Divide the vegetables evenly among four plates. Slice the pork into 1½-inch-thick pieces and top each plate with three or four pieces.

Per Serving
Calorie 292 | Fats 12g| Carbs 15g| Protein 34g

Spicy Peppery Chicken Lettuce Wraps

Prep time: 15 minutes | Cook time: 15 minutes | Serves 2

454 g ground chicken
¼ Teaspoon salt
¼ Teaspoon freshly ground black pepper
3 Tablespoons sesame oil, divided
3 Tablespoon tamari or coconut amino
1 bunch scallions, green and white parts separated
2 tablespoons minced fresh ginger
2 cloves garlic, minced
¼ Teaspoon red pepper flakes
1 medium carrot,

peeled and cut into ¼-inch dice
3 Tablespoons rice vinegar, coconut vinegar, or apple cider vinegar
1 Tablespoon water, plus more as needed
1 head butter lettuce
Sesame seeds, for garnish
Chopped fresh cilantro, for garnish
Sriracha or other hot sauce (optional)
Lime wedges (optional)

1. Season the chicken with the salt and pepper.
2. Heat 1 Tablespoon of the sesame oil in a large skillet or wok over medium-high heat.
3. When it is hot, add the chicken and cook until browned and cooked through, stirring frequently, 3 to 4 minutes.
4. Using a slotted spoon, transfer the cooked chicken to a bowl.
5. Add the soy sauce and stir to combine.
6. Add 1 Tablespoon of the sesame oil and the scallion whites to the pan.
7. Cook, stirring, until the scallions are soft and translucent, about 2 minutes.
8. Add the ginger, garlic, and red pepper flakes and cook until fragrant, 1 minute. Transfer to the bowl with the chicken and toss to combine.
9. Over medium-high heat, add the carrot and vinegar to the pan, which will steam and bubble.
10. Add the water (and more as needed) to cover the carrot dice. Simmer until the carrot is tender and the liquid has evaporated, 3 to 4 minutes.
11. Transfer the mixture to the bowl with the chicken and toss to combine.
12. To serve, separate the head of lettuce into leaves. Top each leaf with the chicken mixture, and then add a sprinkling of the scallion greens, sesame seeds, and cilantro.
13. Serve with sriracha and lime wedges, if you like, as well as extra soy sauce.

Per Serving
Calorie 512| Fats 24g| Carbs 18g| Protein 56g

Garlic Pepper Paleo Chicken Stir Fry

Prep time: 30 minutes | Cook time: 10 minutes | Serves 4

1 Tablespoon and 3/4 Teaspoon low sodium soy sauce
1/2 Teaspoon ground ginger
1/4 Teaspoon crushed red pepper
1/2 Teaspoon salt
3-3/4 cups and 2 tablespoons broccoli florets
1 Tablespoon and 3/4 Teaspoon olive oil
2-1/2 skinless, boneless chicken

breast halves - cut into 1-inch strips
1/3 cup sliced green onions
5 cloves garlic, thinly sliced
1 Tablespoon and 3/4 Teaspoon hoisin sauce
1Tablespoon and 3/4 Teaspoon Chile paste
1/2 Teaspoon black pepper
2 tablespoons and 1/2 Teaspoon chicken stock

1. Place broccoli in a steamer over 1 inch of boiling water, and cover. Cook for about 5 minutes until tender but still firm.
2. In a skillet over medium heat, heat the oil and sauté the chicken, green onions, and garlic until the chicken is no longer pink and juices run clear.
3. Stir the hoisin sauce, Chile paste, and soy sauce into the skillet; season with ginger, red pepper, salt, and black pepper. Stir in the chicken stock and simmer for about 2 minutes.
4. Mix in the steamed broccoli until coated with the sauce mixture.

Per Serving
Calorie 292| Fats 12g| Carbs 15g| Protein 34g

Pegan Grilled Soy Steak and Baby Spinach

Prep time: 15 minutes | Cook time: 30 minutes | Serves 4

For Soy Steak

1 pound flank steak	2 tablespoons soy sauce
⅓ Cup extra-virgin olive oil	½ teaspoon salt
2 cloves garlic, minced	½ teaspoons freshly ground black pepper
3 tablespoons red wine vinegar or apple cider vinegar	½ teaspoon ground cumin

For Baby Spinach Chimichurri

1 bunch fresh cilantro	2 cloves garlic, peeled
1 cup baby spinach	¾ teaspoon red pepper flakes
½ cup extra-virgin olive oil	½ teaspoon ground cumin
3 tablespoons red wine vinegar or apple cider vinegar	Pinch salt

1. In a shallow dish or resealable plastic bag, combine the meat with the oil, garlic, vinegar, and soy sauce.
2. Turn to coat, cover or close, and refrigerate for at least an hour or up to overnight.
3. In a small bowl, mix together the salt, pepper, and cumin and set aside.
4. To make the chimichurri, lop off the cilantro stems with a sharp knife.
5. Add the cilantro leaves to a food processor and pulse a few times to coarsely chop.
6. Add the remaining ingredients and pulse until finely chopped. Alternatively, finely chop all ingredients with a knife and stir to combine.
7. For the steak, set up your grill so there is a direct heat and an indirect heat (cooler) area. Preheat the grill to medium-high heat.
8. Remove the steak from the marinade and gently shake off the excess.
9. Rub the steaks with the salt, pepper, and cumin.
10. Place the steak on the hot side of the grill and sear until browned, about 2 minutes per side.
11. Move the steak to the cooler side of the grill, cover, and continue to cook until the meat is pink in the centre for medium-rare doneness, flipping once, about 6 minutes total, or to your desired degree of doneness.
12. Alternatively, cook the steak in a broiler on high until medium-rare doneness, 4 to 5 minutes per side.
13. Using a sharp or serrated knife, slice the steak against the grain at a steep diagonal angle into 1-inch-thick slices.
14. Divide among four plates and top with the chimichurri.

Per Serving
Calorie 423| Fats 36g| Carbs 2g| Protein 25g

Baked Pork with Vegetables

Prep time: 15 minutes | Cook time: 25 minutes | Serves 4

For Pork

1 pound pork tenderloin	ground black pepper
1 teaspoon salt	1 teaspoon paprika (regular or smoked, optional)
1 teaspoon freshly	

For Vegetables

1 pound Brussels sprouts, trimmed and halved	2 tablespoons extra-virgin olive oil
1 medium yellow or sweet onion, cut into ½-inch wedges	1 teaspoon maple syrup
	1 tablespoon fresh rosemary, minced

1. Preheat the oven to 425°F. Line a baking sheet with aluminum foil or parchment paper.
2. Place the pork in the center of the prepared baking sheet and pat dry. Mix the salt, pepper, and paprika (if using) together in a small bowl.
3. Rub it all over the pork.
4. In a medium bowl, toss the Brussels sprouts and onion with the oil, maple syrup, and rosemary. Spoon the mixture around the pork.
5. Roast the pork and Brussels sprouts until the pork is brown outside and slightly pink inside around 30 minutes.
6. Remove from the oven and let rest for 3 minutes.
7. Divide the vegetables evenly among four plates. Slice the pork into 1½-inch-thick pieces and top each plate with three or four pieces.

Per Serving
Calorie 292| Fats 12g| Carbs 15g| Protein 34g

Juicy Tomato Grass-fed Beef with Pepper

Prep time: 10 minutes | Cook time: 20 minutes | Serves 2

2 red, yellow, orange, or green bell peppers
3 tablespoons extra-virgin olive oil, divided
1 pound ground chicken or ground grass-fed beef
1 tablespoon ground cumin
1 tablespoon chilli powder
1½ teaspoons ground cinnamon
¼ teaspoon salt
¼ teaspoons freshly

ground black pepper
Pinch cayenne pepper (optional)
1 small yellow or sweet onion, diced
2 cloves garlic, minced
6 plum tomatoes, diced, juices reserved
1 cup pitted or pimento-stuffed green olives, quartered
½ cup chopped fresh cilantro

1. Preheat the oven to 400°F.
2. Slice the peppers in half, keeping the stem intact, and remove seeds. Lightly coat with 1 tablespoon olive oil and place on an aluminum foil–lined baking sheet, cut-side up.
3. In a medium bowl, mix the meat with the cumin, chili powder, cinnamon, salt, black pepper, and cayenne (if using).
4. Heat 1 tablespoon of the oil in a large skillet over medium heat. Add the meat and cook until lightly browned but not cooked through, about 2 minutes.
5. Transfer to a bowl using a slotted spoon.
6. In the same skillet, heat the remaining 1 tablespoon oil. Add the onion and cook until soft and translucent, stirring a few times, about 10 minutes.
7. Add the garlic and cook until fragrant, about 30 seconds.
8. Stir in the tomatoes and their juices, olives, and cilantro. Spoon the mixture into the bell pepper halves.
9. Bake until the peppers are tender and any excess tomato juices have evaporated, 10 to 15 minutes.
10. Remove from the oven; allow cooling slightly, and serving.

Per Serving
Calorie 768| Fats 49g| Carbs 29g| Protein 51g

Spaghetti Squash Beef with Black Pepper and Basil

Prep time: 10 minutes | Cook time: 30 minutes | Serves 4

1 (4- to 5-pound) spaghetti squash
1 teaspoon dried oregano
1 teaspoon dried thyme
1 teaspoon onion powder
1 teaspoon garlic powder
½ teaspoon freshly ground black pepper
½ teaspoon red

pepper flakes
¼ teaspoon salt
1 large egg
1 pound grass-fed ground beef (80 per cent lean)
1 pint cherry or grape tomatoes, halved
3 tablespoons extra-virgin olive oil, divided
Torn or chiffonaded fresh basil leaves, for garnish

1. Using a sharp knife carefully slit a few holes in the squash. Microwave on high until tender, about 10 minutes.
2. Preheat the oven to 375°F. Line a rimmed baking sheet with aluminum foil so that it comes up on the sides.
3. In a large bowl, combine all of the spices and the salt.
4. Add the egg and whisk to combine.
5. Add the beef and gently mix until just combined. Do not over mix.
6. Shape the mixture into golf ball–size meatballs (about 16 total) and place on the prepared baking sheet.
7. Toss the tomatoes with 1 tablespoon of the oil and arrange around the meatballs. Bake until just cooked through, 10 to 12 minutes.
8. Slice the squash in half crosswise (see Ingredient Tip), then scoop out and discard the seeds.
9. Use a metal serving spoon or fork to rake the flesh inside the skin into strands and place in a large bowl. Toss with the remaining 2 tablespoons oil.
10. To serve, divide the squash strands evenly among four bowls or plates. Top each with four meatballs.
11. Briefly mix the tomatoes and juices on the baking sheet to make a sauce and carefully pour over the top of each serving.
12. Season with more black pepper, if you like, garnish with basil, and serve.

Per Serving
Calorie 480| Fats 32g| Carbs 30g| Protein 24g

One Pan Pork with apple-onion relish

Prep time: 15 minutes | Cook time: 25 minutes | Serves 2

1½ cups water
½ cup apple cider vinegar
2 tablespoons salt, plus more for seasoning
1 teaspoon freshly ground black pepper (or ½ tablespoon peppercorns), plus more for seasoning
1 teaspoon maple syrup
2 (2-inch-thick) bone-in pastured pork

chops
1 medium red apple
1 teaspoon lemon juice
2 tablespoons unsalted grass-fed butter
1 tablespoon olive oil
1 medium yellow onion, diced
2 cloves garlic, minced
2 tablespoons chopped fresh parsley (optional)

1. In a large shallow bowl, combine the water, vinegar, salt, pepper, and maple syrup and microwave on high until the salt dissolves, about 1 minute.
2. Add the pork, submerging it in the brine. Cover and refrigerate for at least an hour and up to overnight.
3. Place a baking sheet or broiler pan in the oven and set the broiler to high. Remove the chops from the brine, shaking off any excess and patting dry.
4. Season each side evenly with salt and pepper and set aside to dry out further while you prepare the relish.
5. For the relish, dice the apple and toss with the lemon juice.
6. Heat the butter and oil in a medium skillet over medium heat. Add the onion and cook, stirring occasionally, until it starts to caramelize, 7 to 10 minutes.
7. Add the garlic and cook until fragrant, about 30 seconds. Reduce the heat to low, add the apple, stir to coat with the mixture, cover the pan, and cook until just warmed, 1 to 2 minutes.
8. Remove from the heat, stir in the parsley (if using), and set aside.
9. Transfer the pork chops to a baking sheet or broiler pan and broil until slightly pink in the center, about 3 minutes per side, reserving juices from the pan. Let rest for 3 minutes.
10. To serve, divide the chops between two plates. Pour any juice from the pan over the chops, top evenly with the apple-onion relish, and serve.

Per Serving
Calorie 444| Fats 28g| Carbs 25g| Protein 25g

Chicken Paprika with Romesco Sauce

Prep time: 15 minutes | Cook time: 30 minutes | Serves 4

8 small bone-in, skin-on chicken thighs (about 2 pounds)
1 teaspoon paprika (regular or smoked)
1 teaspoon salt
½ teaspoons freshly ground black pepper
Ground turmeric, as needed
4 cups cooked Cauliflower rice
Chopped fresh parsley, for garnish
For Romesco Sauce
1 (12-ounce) jar

roasted red peppers, drained
½ cup extra-virgin olive oil
½ cup raw almonds
3 tablespoons red wine vinegar
1 clove garlic, smashed
1 teaspoon paprika (regular or smoked)
¼ teaspoons freshly ground black pepper
Pinch salt
Pinch cayenne pepper (optional)

1. Preheat the oven to 475°F.
2. Place the chicken thighs on a roasting pan or in a shallow baking dish. Combine the paprika, salt, and pepper in a small bowl, then rub all over the chicken.
3. Bake until fully cooked through, with an internal temperature of 165°F, 25 to 30 minutes.
4. While the chicken bakes, put the Romesco sauce ingredients into a blender or food processor.
5. Process until smooth and thickened. Set aside, or pour into the jar used for the peppers.
6. Sprinkle turmeric over the warm cauliflower rice and stir to color completely. Spoon about 1 cup of the rice onto each plate.
7. Top with two chicken thighs. Pour the pan juices over all.
8. Spread the Romesco sauce on the chicken pieces (or offer on the side), sprinkle with parsley, and serve.

Per Serving
Calorie 817| Fats 66g| Carbs 14g| Protein 48g

Cashew Coconut Chicken with Scallion Greens

Prep time: 15 minutes | Cook time: 20 minutes | Serves 2

2 boneless skinless chicken breasts
3 tablespoons sesame oil, divided
2 cloves garlic, minced, divided
3 tablespoons gluten-free soy sauce, tamari, or coconut amino, divided
3 tablespoons apple cider, rice, or coconut vinegar, divided
2 tablespoons minced

fresh ginger, divided
3 scallions, thinly sliced, green and white parts separated, divided
1 cup raw cashews
1 medium red, orange, or yellow bell pepper, seeded and diced
1 cup snow peas, trimmed
Red pepper flakes, to taste (optional)

1. Cut the chicken breasts into 2-inch strips.
2. In a large shallow bowl, whisk together 1 tablespoon of the sesame oil, half of the garlic, 2 tablespoons of the soy sauce, 2 tablespoons of the vinegar, 1 tablespoon of the ginger, and half of the scallion whites and greens.
3. Add the chicken and turn to coat. Cover and refrigerate for at least 15 minutes while preparing the rest of the stir-fry ingredients, or up to overnight.
4. Heat a dry wok or large skillet over medium-high heat.
5. Add the cashews and cook, stirring, until fragrant and lightly toasted, 1 minute.
6. Remove the cashews from the pan to prevent burning and set aside.
7. Drain the chicken, discarding the marinade, and pat dry. Add 1 tablespoon of the sesame oil to the wok or skillet, still on medium-high heat.
8. When the oil is hot, add the chicken and cook, tossing continuously, until cooked through, about 5 minutes. Transfer to a plate or chopping board.
9. Add the remaining 1 tablespoon sesame oil, the bell pepper, and snow peas and cook, tossing continuously, until tender, about 5 minutes.
10. Add the remaining scallion whites and remaining ginger and cook until just fragrant, about 1 minute.
11. Return the chicken and cashews to the pan.
12. Add the remaining 1 tablespoon soy sauce and vinegar, and the red pepper flakes (if using). Toss to combine.
13. Serve garnished with the reserved scallion greens.

Per Serving
Calorie 774| Fats 49g| Carbs 36g| Protein 49g

Spinach and Berry with Chicken Salad

Prep time: 15 minute | Cook time: 10 minute | Serves 4

4 small beets, peeled and chopped
1 tablespoon plus 1/4 cup olive oil, divided
1 pound boneless, skinless chicken breast
13/4 teaspoons salt, divided
3/4 teaspoon ground black pepper, divided

5 cups baby spinach
1 cup sliced strawberries
1/2 cup chopped pecans
2 tablespoons apple cider vinegar
2 tablespoons maple syrup
2 tablespoons orange juice

1. Place beets in a medium saucepan and cover with water. Boil beets in water until soft, about 20 minutes.
2. Drain beets and allow to cool completely.
3. Meanwhile, heat 1 tablespoon olive oil in a large nonstick frying pan over medium heat.
4. Season both sides of chicken with 3/4 teaspoon salt and 1/4 teaspoon pepper. Add chicken to the pan.
5. Cover the pan and cook until just cooked through, 5–8 minutes on each side. Transfer chicken to a cutting board and let cool.
6. Cut the chicken into bite-sized pieces.
7. In a large bowl, combine chicken, spinach, strawberries, pecans, and cooled beets.
8. In a separate small bowl, whisk together remaining olive oil, vinegar, maple syrup, and orange juice, and pour over salad, tossing well to coat.
9. Season with remaining salt and black pepper.

Per Serving
Calorie 526| Fats 32g| Carbs 22g| Protein 39g

Spicy Ground Chicken with Lime and Soy Sauce

Prep time: 15 minutes | Cook time: 15 minutes | Serves 4

1 pound ground chicken
¼ teaspoon salt
¼ teaspoons freshly ground black pepper
3 tablespoons sesame oil, divided
3 tablespoons gluten-free soy sauce, tamari, or coconut amino, plus more for serving
1 bunch scallions, green and white parts separated
2 tablespoons minced fresh ginger
2 cloves garlic, minced
¼ teaspoon red pepper flakes
1 medium carrot, peeled and cut into ¼-inch dice
3 tablespoons rice vinegar, coconut vinegar, or apple cider vinegar
1 tablespoon water, plus more as needed
1 head butter lettuce
Sesame seeds, for garnish
Chopped fresh cilantro, for garnish
Sriracha or other hot sauce (optional)
Lime wedges (optional)

1. Season the chicken with the salt and pepper.
2. Heat 1 tablespoon of the sesame oil in a large skillet or wok over medium-high heat.
3. When it is hot, add the chicken and cook until browned and cooked through, stirring frequently, 3 to 4 minutes.
4. Using a slotted spoon, transfer the cooked chicken to a bowl. Add the soy sauce and stir to combine.
5. Add 1 tablespoon of the sesame oil and the scallion whites to the pan.
6. Cook, stirring, until the scallions are soft and translucent, about 2 minutes.
7. Add the ginger, garlic, and red pepper flakes and cook until fragrant, 1 minute. Transfer to the bowl with the chicken and toss to combine.
8. Over medium-high heat, add the carrot and vinegar to the pan, which will steam and bubble. Add the water (and more as needed) to cover the carrot dice.
9. Simmer until the carrot is tender and the liquid has evaporated, 3 to 4 minutes. Transfer the mixture to the bowl with the chicken and toss to combine.
10. To serve, separate the head of lettuce into leaves. Top each leaf with the chicken mixture, and then add a sprinkling of the scallion greens, sesame seeds, and cilantro.
11. Serve with sriracha and lime wedges, if you like, as well as extra soy sauce.

Per Serving
Calorie 512| Fats 24g| Carbs 18g| Protein 56g

Pegan Chicken Onion and Carrot Soup

Prep time: 15 minute | Cook time: 30 minute | Serves 6

a small grilled chicken breast or filet of fish for a perfect Pegan meal.
3 tablespoons olive oil
2 pounds carrots, peeled and diced
2 large yellow onions, peeled and diced
2 cloves garlic, peeled and minced
6 cups Basic Vegetable Stock
1 teaspoon minced fresh ginger
Juice and zest from 1 large lemon
1/2 teaspoon ground black pepper
3 green onions, thinly sliced

1. Heat olive oil in a large stockpot over medium heat. Sauté carrots, yellow onions, and garlic until softened, about 5 minutes.
2. Add stock and bring to a boil over high heat. Reduce heat to low and simmer for approximately 25 minutes.
3. Add ginger, lemon juice, and zest. Season with pepper.
4. Garnish with green onions.
5. Serve hot or refrigerate for at least 4 hours.

Per Serving
Calorie 185| Fats 7g| Carbs 29g| Protein 3g

Paleo Chicken Pomegranate Salad

Prep time: 15 minute | Cook time: 30 minute | Serves 4

5 tablespoons olive oil, divided
1 pound boneless, skinless chicken breast
3/4 teaspoon salt
3/4 teaspoon ground black pepper, divided
2 large navel oranges,

peeled and sliced into small pieces
1 large pomegranate, seeds and surrounding flesh only
4 cups arugula
1/2 cup thinly sliced fennel

1. Heat 1 tablespoon olive oil in large nonstick skillet over medium heat. Season both sides of chicken with salt and 1/4 teaspoon pepper.
2. Add chicken to the skillet. Cover and cook until just cooked through, 5–8 minutes on each side.
3. Transfer chicken to a cutting board and let cool. Cut the chicken into bite-sized pieces.
4. Add orange pieces and pomegranate seeds to a large bowl.
5. Add arugula, fennel slices, remaining olive oil, and remaining pepper. Toss to coat and serve immediately.

Per Serving
Calorie 357| Fats 19g| Carbs 21g| Protein 28g

Onion Coconut milk Chicken with almonds

Prep time: 30 minute | Cook time: 20 minute | Serves 4

1 Tablespoon extra-virgin olive oil
1 small yellow onion, diced
2 garlic cloves, grated or minced
¼ Teaspoon salt
¼ Teaspoon freshly ground black pepper
½ Teaspoon curry powder, or more, to taste

½ cup red lentils, rinsed
3 medium carrots, sliced into 1-inch pieces
1½ cups chicken or Veggie Trimmings Stock, or water
1 Can full-fat coconut milk
Crushed almonds, for garnish

1. In a medium saucepan, heat the oil over medium heat.

2. Add the onion and cook until soft and translucent, about 2 minutes.
3. Add the garlic, salt, pepper, and curry powder and cook until fragrant, 30 to 60 seconds.
4. Add the lentils and carrots and pour in the stock and coconut milk. Bring to a boil, reduce the heat, and simmer until the carrots and lentils are soft, about 20 minutes.
5. Serve as it is or purée in a blender or food processor for a creamier consistency, if desired. Garnish with almonds.

Per Serving
Calorie 372 | Fats 28g| Carbs 27g| Protein 9g

Best ever Coconut Chicken Soup with Mushrooms

Prep time: 30 minutes | Cook time: 20 minutes | Serves 6

1 Tablespoon olive oil
1 medium yellow onion, chopped
227 g sliced mushrooms, any variety
Salt and pepper to taste

2 tablespoons fresh minced garlic
1 Teaspoon fresh chopped thyme
1 cup canned coconut milk, whisked
1 cup chicken or vegetable broth

1. Heat the oil in a large saucepan over medium heat.
2. Stir in the onions and mushrooms then season with salt and pepper to taste.
3. Cook for 10 to 12 minutes until the mushroom liquid has cooked off.
4. Stir in the garlic and thyme then whisk in the coconut milk and chicken broth.
5. Bring to a simmer and cook on low heat for 8 to 10 minutes until thick.
6. Remove from heat and puree the soup with an immersion blender – serve hot.

Per Serving
Calorie 200| Fats 15g| Carbs 7.5g| Protein 11g

Chilled Coconut Chicken Avocado Soup

Prep time: 30 minutes | Cook time: 0 minutes | Serves 4

4 ripe avocadoes, pitted and chopped
3 1/2 cups vegetable broth
2/3 cup canned coconut milk

3 small shallots, diced
3 Tablespoons dry white wine
Salt and pepper to taste

1. Combine the avocado, chicken broth and coconut milk in a blender. Blend until smooth and well combined.
2. Add the shallots, wine and salt and pepper – blend smooth.
3. Pour the mixture into a bowl then cover and chill at least 6 hours.
4. Spoon the soup into bowls and garnish with diced avocado and a pinch of cayenne to serve.

Per Serving

Calorie 365| Fats 33g| Carbs 14g| Protein 6g

Super smooth Pumpkin & Ginger Chicken Soup

Prep time: 10 minutes | Cook time: 45 minutes | Serves 5

250 ml coconut milk
60 grams fresh ginger (about 3-4 thumb sized pieces)
1 Teaspoon ground cumin
1 Kilogram pumpkin
500 ml chicken broth or stock

250 ml coconut milk
1/2 Teaspoon ground cinnamon
2 tablespoons coconut oil for roasting the pumpkin
Salt and pepper to taste

1. Preheat oven to 180 C and line a large tray with baking paper.
2. Peel pumpkin and cut into even-sized chunks.
3. Place on tray, drizzle over olive oil and toss around with your hands to coat.
4. Roast pumpkin in the oven for approximately 45 minutes or until super soft and starting to caramelize at the edges.

5. Peel the ginger and gather the rest of the ingredients while the pumpkin is roasting.
6. Place cooked pumpkin, chicken broth/ stock, coconut milk, ginger, cumin and cinnamon into blender jug.
7. Blend until super smooth. Season it with salt and pepper to taste.
8. Heat a portion of the soup in a saucepan over the stove, to serve (or microwave the soup if that's more convenient for you). Enjoy!

Per Serving

Calorie 372| Fats 28g| Carbs27 g| Protein9 g

Paleo Lean Beef Vegetables Soup

Prep time: 15 minute | Cook time: 20 minute | Serves 14

1 pound 85% lean ground beef
1 small head cabbage, cored and chopped
2 green onions, chopped
1 medium red bell pepper, seeded and chopped
1 medium bunch celery, chopped
1 cup chopped carrots
4 cups Basic Vegetable Stock (see

recipe in this chapter)
4 cups water
3 cloves garlic, peeled and minced
1/4 teaspoon crushed red pepper flakes
1/4 teaspoon dried basil
1/4 teaspoon dried oregano
1/4 teaspoon dried thyme
1/4 teaspoon onion powder

1. Heat a large skillet over medium-high heat. Add beef and cook, breaking up the lumps, until the meat is cooked through and just beginning to brown, 8–10 minutes. Drain excess fat.
2. Place beef, cabbage, green onions, bell pepper, celery, and carrots in a 6-quart slow cooker.
3. Pour in stock and water.
4. Stir in garlic, pepper flakes, basil, oregano, thyme, and onion powder. Cover and cook on low for 8–10 minutes.

Per Serving

Calorie 107| Fats 5g| Carbs 8g| Protein 8g

CHAPTER 12: PEGAN SEA FOOD RECIPES

Peppery Shrimp and Steak for Two

Prep time: 30 minutes | Cook time: 25 minutes | Serves 2

12 medium shrimp, peeled and deveined
2 filet mignon steaks
2 Teaspoons olive oil
1 Tablespoon butter, melted
1 Tablespoon finely minced onion
1 Teaspoon steak seasoning
1 Tablespoon finely minced onion
1 Tablespoon white wine
1 Teaspoon Worcestershire sauce
1 Teaspoon seafood seasoning
1/8 Teaspoon freshly ground black pepper
1 Teaspoon lemon juice
1 Teaspoon dried parsley

1. In a bowl, whisk 1 Tablespoon olive oil, onion, butter, Worcestershire sauce, wine, lemon juice, parsley, seafood seasoning, garlic, and black pepper together
2. Toss to coat evenly. Cover bowl with plastic wrap and refrigerate for flavors to blend, at least 15 minutes.
3. Preheat an outdoor grill for medium-high heat and lightly oil the grate. Coat steaks with 2 Teaspoons olive oil; sprinkle with steak seasoning.
4. Cook steaks until they are beginning to firm and have reached your desired doneness, 5 to 7 minutes per side.
5. Transfer steaks to a platter and loosely tent with a piece of aluminum foil.
6. Remove shrimp from marinade and grill until they are bright pink on the outside and the meat is no longer transparent in the canter, 2 to 3 minutes per side.

Per Serving
Calorie 444| Fats 34.5g| Carbs 2.7g| Protein 9g

Avocado Nori with Pickled Ginger

Prep time: 15 minutes | Cook time: 30 minutes | Serves 2

2 sheets sushi nori
1 medium avocado, pitted and peeled
2 tablespoons sesame seeds, divided (optional)
113 g smoked salmon (about 4 thin slices)
1 medium cucumber,
cut into matchsticks
3 Tablespoons pickled ginger (optional)
1 Teaspoon wasabi paste (optional)
Gluten-free soy sauce, tamari, or coconut amino, for dipping

1. Lay 1 piece of nori on a sheet of parchment paper or aluminium foil on a flat surface.
2. In a small bowl, mash the avocado with a fork.
3. Spread half of the avocado mixture on the nori sheet, leaving a ½-inch strip uncovered along the top edge.
4. Sprinkle 1 Tablespoon of the sesame seeds (if using), evenly over the avocado. Arrange 2 pieces of the smoked salmon horizontally, covering the avocado.
5. Arrange the cucumber horizontally, running up the length of the sheet and creating columns to cover the salmon.
6. Wet the tip of your finger and run it along the exposed seam. Roll the nori tightly away from you, using the foil as a guide and pressing firmly to seal.
7. Repeat the process with the remaining nori sheet and ingredients, and refrigerate both for at least 30 minutes to firm up.
8. Using a very sharp or serrated knife, slice each roll into 6 to 8 pieces.
9. Serve with pickled ginger and wasabi (if using) and soy sauce for dipping.

Per Serving
Calorie 487 | Fats 32g| Carbs 26g| Protein 28g

Creamy Salmon Capers with Spiralled Zoodles

Prep time: 30 minutes | Cook time: 5 minutes | Serves 2

A small shallot, chopped
1 Tablespoon of almond flour
1 cup sour cream
1/2 cup parmesan
1/3 cup sliced mushrooms of your choice
1 cup broccoli florets
1 Tablespoon capers
1 Tablespoon chopped chives

2 tablespoons s chopped parsley
2 fillets of wild Alaskan salmon
1 Tablespoon avocado oil
3 Tablespoon s pastured butter
2 cloves of garlic, minced
Lemon juice to taste
Black pepper to taste

1. Descale and wash the fish. Fry the salmon with the avocado oil for a few minutes, turning once (do not overcook).
2. Remove its skin and eat it. Add lemon juice on the fish, and set aside.
3. Heat water in a small water and add the mushrooms to boil for a few minutes.
4. Add the broccoli florets for another 1-2 minutes (must remain a little bit crunchy). Strain, set aside.
5. In a large pot heat the butter with the black pepper, garlic and shallot.
6. Add the sour cream and parmesan when browned. Stir to combine, but don't let it get too cooked (no more than 30 seconds on fire, just enough for the parmesan to melt).
7. Cut the salmon in small pieces, add it to the cream.
8. Add the mushrooms, broccoli, and capers, and carefully combine.
9. Sprinkle with chives or parsley; serve with spiralled "zoodles".

Per Serving
Calorie 216.9| Fats 10.9g| Carbs 5.8g| Protein 24g

One pan Broiled Salmon with Yellow Miso

Prep time: 25 minutes | Cook time: 10 minutes | Serves 2

2 salmon fillets
¼ cup white or yellow miso
2 tablespoons rice or coconut vinegar
2 tablespoons sesame oil, divided
1 Tablespoon gluten-free soy sauce, tamari, or coconut amino
1 Tablespoon minced fresh ginger
1 clove garlic, minced

680 g (medium bunch) baby bok choy, core removed, sliced into 1½-inch pieces, white stem and leafy green parts separated
2 tablespoons thinly sliced scallion whites (optional)
2 tablespoons thinly sliced scallion greens, for garnish (optional)

1. Heat the broiler to high.
2. On a baking sheet or broiler pan, place the salmon, skin-side down, and pat it dry.
3. In a small bowl, whisk together the miso, vinegar, 1 Tablespoon of the sesame oil, the soy sauce, ginger, and garlic.
4. Spread 2 tablespoons of the glaze evenly over the top of the salmon, setting aside the remainder. Let it stand for 10 minutes, if you have time.
5. Broil the salmon until the glaze is bubbly, 3 to 4 minutes. Cover it loosely with foil and continue to broil until slightly pink in the center, another 3 to 4 minutes.
6. Remove the salmon from the broiler, remove the foil, and let it cool.
7. In a large skillet over medium-high heat, heat the remaining 1 Tablespoon sesame oil.
8. Add the bok choy stems and scallion whites (if using) and cook until just tender, 2 to 3 minutes.
9. Stir in the remaining miso glaze and cook until fragrant, 30 to 60 seconds.
10. Add the bok choy greens, cover, and steam until just wilted, 30 seconds. Toss to coat with the sauce.
11. To serve, divide the bok choy evenly between two plates.
12. Top each with a salmon fillet and sprinkle with scallion greens (if using).

Per Serving
Calorie 602| Fats 36g| Carbs 20g| Protein 45g

Garlic and Herb Mussels in Rose Broth

Prep time: 18 minutes | Cook time: 10 minutes | Serves 4

32 ounce mussels
1 Tablespoon extra-virgin olive oil
2 shallots, minced
3 cloves garlic, minced
2 cups chicken or Veggie Trimmings Stock
¼ cup lemon juice (from 2 lemons)
¼ cup chopped fresh parsley, plus more for garnish
¼ cup chopped fresh dill (optional)

3 Tablespoons chopped fresh thyme
½ Teaspoon salt
¼ Teaspoon freshly ground black pepper
¼ Teaspoon red pepper flakes (optional)
3 cups baby spinach (or spinach leaves torn into smaller pieces)
2 tablespoons cold unsalted grass-fed butter, cubed

1. Rinse the mussels under cold running water, pulling off their black beards as needed. Place in a strainer to drain and set aside.
2. Heat the oil in a large, deep skillet, stockpot, or Dutch oven over medium-high heat.
3. Add the shallots and cook, stirring, until soft and translucent, about 2 minutes. Add the garlic and cook until fragrant, 30 seconds.
4. Add the stock, lemon juice, herbs, salt, pepper, and red pepper flakes (if using), and stirring to combine. Bring the stock to a boil.
5. Add the mussels, cover, and cook, undisturbed, until the mussels open their shells, about 5 minutes.
6. Reduce the heat to low. Discard any mussels that have not yet opened. Divide the mussels among four large serving bowls.
7. Add the spinach to the broth, cover, and cook until just wilted, 1 to 2 minutes. Remove the lid and turn off the heat. Let sit for 1 minute, then add the cold butter, one piece at a time, stirring in each one until fully melted before adding the next one.
8. Spoon the broth over the mussels in the bowls, garnish with more parsley if you like, and serve.

Per Serving
Calorie 342| Fats 16g| Carbs 17g| Protein 13g

Spicy Crabs with Chilled Coleslaw Mix

Prep time: 17 minutes | Cook time: 30 minutes | Serves 2

1 package shredded coleslaw mix
Grated zest and juice of 1 medium lemon
Grated zest of 1 medium navel orange
2 tablespoons Dijon mustard
2 large eggs
1 Tablespoon Dijon mustard
½ Teaspoon sea salt
½ Teaspoon Old Bay seasoning or paprika

¼ Teaspoon freshly ground black pepper
1 can cooked jumbo lump crab meat, drained and patted dry
¾ cup cooled or chilled cooked Easy Cauliflower Rice, mashed with a fork
2 tablespoons chopped fresh parsley
2 tablespoons extra-virgin olive oil

1. To make the slaw, toss the coleslaw mix with the lemon zest and juice, orange zest, and mustard in a large bowl until evenly coated.
2. Refrigerate it for at least 30 minutes.
3. In a medium bowl, whisk together the eggs, mustard, salt, Old Bay seasoning, and pepper.
4. Fold in the crab, cauliflower rice, and parsley until well combined. Refrigerate until slightly firm, about 10 minutes.
5. Remove the crab mixture from the refrigerator and form into four patties about 2 inches thick and 3 inches in diameter.
6. Heat the olive oil in a large skillet or cast-iron pan over medium-high heat. When the oil is hot, add two of the crab cakes.
7. Cook until golden brown, about 3 minutes per side. Transfer to a paper towel–lined plate. Repeat with the remaining cakes.
8. Place two crab cakes on each plate and serve with the chilled slaw.

Per Serving
Calorie 438| Fats 21g| Carbs 15g| Protein 52g

Best Tuna Grape Salad

Prep time: 10 minutes | Cook time: 5 minutes | Serves 4

1/2 stalk of celery
5-6 grapes
1 good quality tuna
1 Tablespoon of mayo

1 Tablespoon Black pepper
1 romaine lettuce

1. Drain the tuna, and place on a bowl. Cut into smaller pieces using your hands.
2. Wash the celery and grapes, and cut them very thinly.
3. Add them to the bowl.
4. Add the mayo, black pepper, and mix well using a spoon.
5. Serve on romaine lettuce leaves, or refrigerate for up to 1 day.

Per Serving

Calorie 170| Fats 7g| Carbs 4g| Protein 20g

Easy Butter Shrimp Scampi with Parsley Leaves

Prep time: 15 minutes | Cook time: 10 minutes | Serves 3

454 g jumbo shrimp (about 12), peeled and deveined
3 Tablespoons extra-virgin olive oil, divided
6 cloves garlic, minced
1 cup unsalted chicken broth or stock
Grated zest and juice from
1 medium lemon
½ Teaspoon red pepper flakes, or to taste

¼ Teaspoon sea salt or Himalayan salt, or to taste
½ Teaspoon freshly ground black pepper, or to taste
¼ cup (½ stick) cold unsalted grass-fed butter, cubed
8 cups baby spinach leaves
2 to 3 Tablespoons chopped fresh parsley (optional)

1. Pat the shrimp very dry with paper towels. Heat 2 tablespoons of the olive oil in a large skillet over medium-high heat.
2. Add the shrimp and cook until pink, flipping once, about 2 minutes per side. Transfer to a large bowl or plate. 2
3. Reduce the heat to medium and add remaining 1 Tablespoon oil. Add the garlic and cook until just fragrant, about 1 minute.

4. Add the broth, lemon zest and juice, red pepper flakes, salt, and black pepper, increase the heat to medium-high, and bring to a simmer.
5. Reduce the sauce by half, scraping up any browned bits from the bottom with a wooden spoon, about 5 minutes.
6. Remove the pan from the heat and allow cooling slightly. Add butter, one cube at a time, stirring continually with a wooden spoon until the sauce thickens.
7. To serve, divide spinach evenly among four plates. Top each plate with about 4 shrimp. Divide the sauce evenly among the plates and garnish with the parsley.

Per Serving

Calorie 644 | Fats 46g| Carbs 9g| Protein 53g

Garlicky Fish Fillets with Parsley leaves

Prep time: 30 minutes | Cook time: 30 minutes | Serves 4

2 skinless Arctic char or other whitefish fillets
1 Teaspoon kosher salt
1 Teaspoon freshly ground black pepper
½ cup extra-virgin olive oil

3 cloves garlic, minced
¾ cup fresh parsley leaves, minced, divided
¼ cup grated lemon zest (from 6 small or 4 large lemons), divided

1. Place the fish fillets lengthwise in a 13-by-9-inch baking dish and season with the salt and pepper on both sides.
2. In a small bowl, whisk together the olive oil, garlic, half of the parsley, and half of the lemon zest. Pour evenly over the fish, cover, and marinate in the refrigerator for at least 30 minutes and up to overnight.
3. Preheat the oven to 350°F. 3. Bake the fish until just cooked through, 15 to 20 minutes.
4. Cut each fillet into 2 pieces, top evenly with the remaining parsley and lemon zest, and serve with Lemony Sautéed Chard with Red Onion and Herbs or another vegetable side or salad.

Per Serving

Calorie 216.9 | Fats 10.9g| Carbs 5.8g| Protein 24g

Creamy Zucchini Clam Shallow Bowls

Prep time: 10 minute | Cook time: 20 minute | Serves 4

2 medium zucchini
2 tablespoons extra-virgin olive oil
4 cloves garlic, minced
4 (6-ounce) cans chopped clams
½ teaspoon red pepper flakes
¼ cup (½ stick) cold

unsalted grass-fed butter, cubed
2 teaspoons grated lemon zest
Chopped fresh parsley, for garnish
Freshly ground black pepper
2 lemon wedges, for garnish (optional)

1. Using a spiralized, cut the zucchini into noodles or use purchased zoodles (thaw if frozen). Set aside.
2. In a large, deep skillet over medium-high heat, heat olive oil and garlic until fragrant, 1 to 2 minutes, taking care that the garlic doesn't brown.
3. Drain the liquid from clams into the skillet, leaving the clams in the cans. Add the red pepper flakes. Bring to a simmer and cook until the liquid is reduced to ¾ cup, about 15 minutes.
4. Add the clams to the broth and cook until heated through, about 1 minute. Turn off the heat and let sit for 1 minute.
5. Add the butter, stirring in each cube until fully melted before adding the next one. Stir in the lemon zest. Add zucchini noodles and toss to coat.
6. To serve, divide between four plates or shallow bowls. Top with parsley and black pepper, and serve with lemon wedges, if desired.

Easy Bacon & Shrimp Salmon Recipe

Prep time: 30 minute | Cook time: 15 minute | Serves 4

4 ounces smoked salmon, sliced off
4 ounces shrimp, deveined
1 mug mushrooms, sliced

4 bacon slices, sliced off
Table salt and black pepper to the taste
½ mug coconut cream

1. Heat a dish over moderate heat, insert bacon, Prepare and shake for 5 minutes.
2. Insert mushrooms, prepare and shake for 5 minutes longer.
3. Insert salmon, prepare and shake for 3 minutes.
4. Insert fish and prepare for two minutes.
5. Insert pepper, table salt and coconut cream, shake fry 1 minute, eliminate heat and split between dishes.

Shrimp Lettuce Garden Salad

Prep time: 15 minute | Cook time: 15 minute | Serves 6

1 head romaine lettuce- rinsed, dried and chopped
2 bunches radishes, sliced
1 bunch green onions, chopped

1 cucumber, cleaned and chopped
3 tomatoes, chopped
3 stalks celery, chopped
1 (4.5 ounce) can small shrimp, drained

1. In a large bowl, combine the Romaine, radishes, green onions, cucumber, tomatoes, celery and shrimp.
2. Toss with favourite salad dressing and serve.

Homemade Shrimp and Onions with Grits

Prep time: 10 minute | Cook time: 25 minute | Serves 4

1 lb. medium shrimp
1/8 onion, diced
1/2 cup butter
1 tablespoon garlic salt (or 1 garlic clove finely chopped)

1 tablespoon salt
1/2 tablespoon pepper
1/2 bell pepper (green)

1. Shell, clean and devein shrimp. Remove tails. Sprinkle with seasonings.
2. Melt butter in large skillet.
3. Add shrimp, bell pepper and onion and garlic if using. Cook over medium heat for 3-5 minutes.
4. Move skillet from side to side to keep onions moving and to discourage sticking. Watch closely. Do not overcook nor scorch onions.
5. Serve over white rice or grits.

Shrimp Coconut Chicken Soup

Prep time: 30 minute | Cook time: 10 minute | Serves 2

¼ mug coconut amino
5 ounces canned bamboo shoots, sliced
Black pepper to the taste
¼ tsp. fish sauce
1-pound shrimp, peeled and deveined
½ pound snow peas

4 scallions, sliced off
1 and ½ Tablespoon coconut oil
1 small ginger root, finely sliced off
8 mugs chicken stock
1 tablespoon sesame oil
½ tablespoon chili oil

1. Warm up a pot with the coconut oil over moderate heat, insert scallions and ginger, shake and prepare for 2 minutes.
2. Insert coconut amino, stock, black pepper and fish sauce, shake and bring to a boil.
3. Insert shrimp, snow peas and bamboo shoots, shake and prepare for 3 minutes.
4. Insert sesame oil and warm chilli oil, shake, distribute into pots and serve.

Baked Salmon with Lemon Caper Butter Recipe

Prep time: 30 minute | Cook time: 25 minute | Serves 2

2 (5 ounce) salmon fillets
Kosher salt and pepper
4 lemon slices
Non-stick spray
3 tablespoons unsalted butter
2 cloves garlic,

minced
2 tablespoons capers drained and rinsed
1/2 teaspoon lemon zest
Juice of 1/2 of a lemon
Kosher salt and fresh cracked pepper

1. Preheat oven to 450 degrees.
2. Line a baking sheet with aluminum foil and spray with non-stick spray.
3. Place salmon fillets on the prepared baking sheet.
4. Sprinkle fillets with kosher salt and fresh cracked pepper. Place 2 lemon slices on top of each fillet. Bake for 10 minutes.
5. Remove and tent with aluminum foil for 10 more minutes. Fish will continue to cook during this time. It will flake easily when done.

6. While salmon is cooking, in a small sauce pan, melt butter over medium heat.
7. Add garlic, capers, and lemon zest and lemon juice. Cook for 2 minutes. Season to taste with salt and pepper.
8. Remove lemon slices and discard. Gently slide a turner or serving spatula between the skin and the flesh of the fillet to remove the skin, it should separate very easily.
9. Transfer fillet to a serving platter and spoon lemon caper butter over the top. Serve

One Pan Rainbow Butter Trout with Lemon

Prep time: 15 minute | Cook time: 10 minute | Serves 2

1 whole rainbow trout fileted and pin-boned
Kosher salt
Fresh lemon juice to taste
1 teaspoon chopped fresh parsley
2 tablespoons mixed capers made from plant buds like dandelions,

nasturtiums, chives, spruce
2 tablespoons clarified unsalted butter or ghee
1 tablespoon unsalted butter chilled
1/4 cup chicken stock
All-purpose flour as needed for dredging the fish

1. Heat a large sauté pan with the clarified butter.
2. Season the trout filets with salt and pepper, then dredge in the all-purpose flour.
3. Add the trout skin side down to the pan and cook until lightly browned and crisp.
4. Flip the trout filets quickly to cook the flesh side, then remove and keep warm on a pre-heated dinner plate.
5. Add the capers to the pan, and then deglaze the pan with the stock.
6. Season the sauce to taste with lemon juice, then whisk in the cold, unsalted butter to form a creamy sauce, keeping the pan on medium-high and whisking constantly.
7. Double check the seasoning for salt to taste, then spoon over the fish and serve immediately.

Chicken Mushroom Shrimp Mix with Green Onions

Prep time: 30 minute | Cook time: 20 minute | Serves 4

½ pound mushrooms, roughly sliced off
Table salt and black pepper to the taste
¼ mug mayonnaise
2 Tablespoon sriracha
½ tsp. paprika
¼ tsp. xanthan gum
1 green onion stalk, sliced off
20 shrimp, raw, peeled and deveined

2 chicken breasts, boneless and skinless
2 handfuls spinach leaves
2 teaspoons lime juice
1 tablespoon coconut oil
½ tsp. red pepper, crushed
1 tsp. garlic grinding grains

1. Warm up a dish with the oil over moderate gigantic warmth, embed chicken bosoms, season with table salt, pepper, red pepper and garlic pounding grains, plan for 8 minutes, flip and get ready for 6 minutes more.
2. Supplement mushrooms, more table salt and pepper and plan for a couple of moments.
3. Warm up another dish over moderate warmth, embed shrimp, sriracha, paprika, xanthan and mayo, shake and get ready until shrimp turn pink.
4. Eliminate heat, embed lime squeeze and shake everything.
5. Serve spinach on plates, appropriate chicken and mushroom, top with shrimp consolidate, decorate with green onions.

Salmon Avocado Coconut Milk Soup

Prep time: 30 minute | Cook time: 20 minute | Serves 4

2 garlic cloves, chopped
6 mugs chicken stock
1-pound salmon, slice into small pieces
2 teaspoons thyme, dried
4 leeks, trimmed and

sliced
Table salt and black pepper to the taste
2 Tablespoon avocado oil
1 and ¾ mugs coconut milk

1. Warm up a pot with the oil over moderate heat, insert leeks and garlic, shake and prepare for 5 minutes.

2. Insert thyme, stock, table salt and pepper, shake and simmer for 15 minutes.
3. Insert coconut milk and salmon, shake and bring to a simmer again. Distribute into pots and serve right away.

Chicken and Shrimp Skillet

Prep time: 15 minute | Cook time: 30 minute | Serves 4

½ pound chicken, sliced thin
1 pound (16-20) extra-large shrimp, cleaned
2 tablespoons olive oil
1 tablespoon unsalted butter
1 cup diced white onion

2 cloves garlic, chopped
¾ cup short grain white rice, rinsed
3 cups chicken stock
Salt and pepper
Fresh parsley, for garnish
Lemon slices, for garnish

1. Slice chicken into thin 2-inch strips. Peel shrimp, leaving the tail on, and clean shrimp by running a paring knife down the back and rinsing out the shrimp vein with cold water.
2. In a large skillet, add 2 tablespoons olive oil over medium heat. Add chicken. Season chicken with a pinch of salt and pepper and cook for 6 minutes until chicken is cooked through
3. Remove chicken from skillet. Add butter, onion, and garlic. Cook for 3-4 minutes, until vegetables are soft.
4. Add rinsed rice to skillet and pour in chicken stock. Stir together and bring mixture to a simmer.
5. Turn heat down to low. Add chicken back to mixture, cover, and cook for 15 minutes on low heat.
6. After simmering for 15 minutes, add cleaned shrimp to skillet. Cover and cook for another 5 minutes.
7. Uncover skillet and taste rice. Season with salt and pepper if needed. If the skillet has too much liquid, cook uncovered for a minute to thicken.
8. Finish chicken and shrimp skillet by garnishing with fresh parsley and lemon slices. Serve skillet while warm.

Shrimp Cucumber Noodles with Chili Sauce

Prep time: 30 minute | Cook time: 20 minute | Serves 4

Table salt and black pepper to the taste
1 tablespoon stevia
2 teaspoons fish sauce
1 cucumber
½ mug basil, sliced off

½ pound shrimp, already prepared, peeled and deveined
2 Tablespoon lime juice
2 teaspoons chilli garlic sauce

1. Put cucumber noodles on a paper towel, wrap up with another one and press well.
2. Put into a pot and combine with basil, shrimp, table salt and pepper.
3. In another pot, combine stevia with fish sauce, lime juice and chili sauce and whisk well.
4. Insert this to shrimp salad, fling to coat well and serve.

Baked Garlic marinade Arctic char Fillets

Prep time: 30 minute | Cook time: 20 minute | Serves 4

2 (¾-pound) skinless Arctic char or other whitefish fillets
1 teaspoon kosher salt
1 teaspoon freshly ground black pepper
½ cup extra-virgin olive oil

3 cloves garlic, minced
¾ cup fresh parsley leaves, minced, divided
¼ cup grated lemon zest (from 6 small or 4 large lemons), divided

1. Place the fish fillets lengthwise in a 13-by-9-inch baking dish and season with the salt and pepper on both sides.
2. In a small bowl, whisk together the olive oil, garlic, half of the parsley, and half of the lemon zest.
3. Pour evenly over the fish, cover, and marinate in the refrigerator for at least 30 minutes and up to overnight.
4. Preheat the oven to 350°F.
5. Bake the fish until just cooked through, 15 to 20 minutes.
6. Cut each fillet into 2 pieces, top evenly with the remaining parsley and lemon zest and serve.

Classic Shrimp Creole Recipe

Prep time: 30 minute | Cook time: 15 minute | Serves 4

Juice of 1 lemon
Table salt and black pepper to the taste
1 tsp. Creole seasoning

½ pound big shrimp, peeled and deveined
2 teaspoons Worcestershire sauce
2 teaspoons olive oil

1. Organize shrimp in one layer in a baking dish, season with table salt and pepper and drizzle the oil.
2. Insert Worcestershire sauce, lemon juice and Garnish Creole seasoning.
3. Fling shrimp a bit, introduce in the oven, set it on the broiler and prepare for 10 minutes.
4. Distribute between 2 plates and serve.

Creamy Coconut Shrimp Vegetable Pot

Prep time: 20 minute | Cook time: 20 minute | Serves 4

¼ mug red pepper, roasted and sliced off
14 ounces canned tomatoes, sliced off
¼ mug cilantro, sliced off
2 Tablespoon sriracha sauce
¼ mug yellow onion, sliced off
¼ mug olive oil

1 garlic clove, chopped
1 and ½ pounds shrimp, peeled and deveined
1 mug coconut milk
Table salt and black pepper to the taste
2 Tablespoon lime juice

1. Warm up a dish with the oil over moderate heat, insert onion, shake and prepare for 4 minutes.
2. Insert peppers and garlic, shake and prepare for 4 minutes more.
3. Insert cilantro, tomatoes and shrimp, shake and prepare until shrimp turn pink.
4. Insert coconut milk and sriracha sauce, shake and bring to a gentle simmer.
5. Insert table salt, pepper and lime juice, shake, shift to pots and serve.

Homemade Shrimp Bamboo Shoots Pot

Prep time: 20 minute | Cook time: 20 minute | Serves 4

¼ mug coconut amino
5 ounces canned bamboo shoots, sliced
Black pepper to the taste
¼ tsp. fish sauce
1-pound shrimp, peeled and deveined
½ pound snow peas

4 scallions, sliced off
1 and ½ Tablespoon coconut oil
1 small ginger root, finely sliced off
8 mugs chicken stock
1 tablespoon sesame oil
½ tablespoon chili oil

1. Warm up a pot with the coconut oil over moderate heat, insert scallions and ginger, shake and prepare for 2 minutes.
2. Insert coconut amino, stock, black pepper and fish sauce, shake and bring to a boil.
3. Insert shrimp, snow peas and bamboo shoots, shake and prepare for 3 minutes.
4. Insert sesame oil and warm chili oil, shake, distribute into pots and serve.

Baked Barramundi Tomato Recipe

Prep time: 30 minute | Cook time: 20 minute | Serves 4

2 barramundi fillets
¼ mug black olives, sliced off
1 tablespoon lemon zest
2 Tablespoon lemon zest
Table salt and black pepper to the taste
2 tsp. olive oil

2 teaspoons Italian seasoning
¼ mug green olives, pitted and sliced off
¼ mug cherry tomatoes, sliced off
2 Tablespoon parsley, sliced off
1 tablespoon olive oil

1. Rub fish with table salt, pepper, Italian seasoning and 2 teaspoons olive oil, shift to a baking dish and leave aside for now.
2. Meanwhile, in a pot, combine tomatoes with all the olives, table salt, pepper, lemon zest and lemon juice, parsley and 1 tablespoon olive oil and fling everything well.
3. Introduce fish in the oven at 400 degrees F and bake for 12 minutes.
4. Distribute fish on plates, top with tomato relish and serve.

Instant Pepper Shrimp Snap Pea Curry

Prep time: 30 minute | Cook time: 15 minute | Serves 2

1 tablespoon olive oil
½ mug cilantro, sliced off
1 tablespoon garlic, chopped
½ mug green onion, sliced off
½ tsp. red pepper flakes
1-pound shrimp, peeled and deveined
Table salt and black

pepper to the taste
4 cherry tomatoes, sliced off
2 mugs sugar snap peas, sliced lengthwise
1 red bell pepper, slice
10 ounces coconut milk
2 Tablespoon lime juice

1. Warm up a dish with the oil over moderate immense heat, insert snap peas and shake-fry for 2 minutes.
2. Insert pepper and prepare for 3 minutes more. Insert cilantro, garlic, green onions and pepper flakes, shake and prepare for 3 minute.
3. Insert tomatoes and coconut milk, shake and simmer everything for 5 minutes.
4. Insert shrimp and lime juice, shake and prepare for 5 minutes. Season with table salt and pepper, shake and serve warm.

Simple Lemon Garlic Shrimp Bowl

Prep time: 30 minute | Cook time: 20 minute | Serves 4

2 Tablespoon lemon juice
2 Tablespoon garlic, chopped
1 tablespoon lemon zest

2 Tablespoon olive oil
1 tablespoon ghee
1-pound shrimp, peeled and deveined
Table salt and black pepper to the taste

1. Warm up a dish with the oil and the ghee over moderate immense heat, insert shrimp and prepare for 2 minutes.
2. Insert garlic, shake and prepare for 4 minutes more.
3. Insert lemon juice, lemon zest, table salt and pepper, shake, remove heat and serve.

Classic Cashew Salmon Recipe

Prep time: 15 minute | Cook time: 15 minute | Serves 3

1 lb. wild salmon fillets	mustard
1 tsp. honey	Pinch of salt
1 tsp. whole-grain	3 Tbsp. (1 oz.) cashews

1. Preheat broiler to high heat. Line a baking sheet with foil, and lay salmon on it skin side down.
2. In a small bowl, stir together honey, mustard, and salt. Spread mixture evenly on fish.
3. In a small bowl, stir together honey, mustard, and salt. Spread mixture evenly on fish.
4. Use the back of a wooden spoon or the side of a chef's knife to crush cashews. Sprinkle over salmon.
5. Broil until salmon flakes easily with a fork in the thickest part, which can take 5–10 minutes depending on your broiler and the thickness of the fillet.

Homemade Salmon Oregano Skewers

Prep time: 15 minute | Cook time: 10 minute | Serves 4

2 Tablespoon chopped fresh oregano	into 1-inch pieces
2 tsp sesame seeds	2 lemons, very thinly sliced into rounds
1 tsp ground cumin	olive oil cooking spray
1/4 tsp crushed red pepper flakes	1 tsp kosher salt
1-1/2 pounds skinless wild salmon fillet, cut	16 bamboo skewers soaked in water

1. Heat the grill on medium heat and spray the grates with oil.
2. Mix oregano, sesame seeds, cumin, and red pepper flakes in a small bowl to combine; set spice mixture aside.
3. Beginning and ending with salmon, thread salmon and folded lemon slices onto 8 pairs of parallel skewers to make 8 kebabs total.
4. Spray the fish lightly with oil and season kosher salt and the reserved spice mixture.
5. Grill the fish, turning occasionally, until fish is opaque throughout, about 8 to 10 minutes total.

Flounder Fillets with Celery Shrimp Stuffing

Prep time: 15 minute | Cook time: 20 minute | Serves 6

For Stuffing

6 tablespoons butter, cubed	shrimp, peeled, deveined and chopped
1 small onion, finely chopped	1/4 cup beef broth
1/4 cup finely chopped celery	1 teaspoon diced pimientos, drained
1/4 cup finely chopped green pepper	1 teaspoon Worcestershire sauce
1 pound uncooked	1/2 teaspoon dill weeds

For Fish

6 flounder fillets (3 ounces each)	1 teaspoon minced fresh parsley
5 tablespoons butter, melted	1/2 teaspoon paprika
2 tablespoons lemon juice	Salt and pepper to taste

1. Preheat oven to 375°. In a large skillet, melt butter. Add onion, celery and green pepper; sauté until tender.
2. Add shrimp; cook and stir until shrimp turn pink.
3. Add broth, pimientos, Worcestershire sauce, dill, chives, salt and cayenne; heat through. Remove from heat; stir in bread crumbs. Spoon about 1/2 cup stuffing onto each fillet; roll up.
4. Place seam side down in a greased 13x9-in. baking dish. Drizzle with butter and lemon juice.
5. Sprinkle with seasonings. Bake, uncovered, 20-25 minutes or until fish flakes easily with a fork.

Basil Butter Shrimp

Prep time: 20 minute | Cook time: 30 minute | Serves 9

2 ½ tablespoons olive oil
¼ cup butter, melted
1 ½ lemons, juiced
3 tablespoons Dijon mustard
½ cup minced fresh basil leaves

3 cloves garlic, minced
Salt to taste
White pepper
3 pounds fresh shrimp, peeled and deveined
Skewers

1. In a shallow, non-porous dish or bowl, mix together olive oil and melted butter. Stir in lemon juice, mustard, basil, and garlic, and season with salt and white pepper.
2. Add shrimp, and toss to coat. Cover, and refrigerate for 1 hour.
3. Preheat grill to high heat. Remove shrimp from marinade, and thread onto skewers. Discard marinade.
4. Lightly oil grill grate, and arrange skewers on preheated grill. Cook for 4 minutes, turning once, or until opaque.

Cheesy Garlic Tuna Cakes Recipe

Prep time: 10 minute | Cook time: 10 minute | Makes 8 cakes

2 5 oz. cans of tuna in water well drained
3 garlic cloves grated
1/4 cup finely chopped white onion
1/4 teaspoon salt
1/4 teaspoon black pepper
1 teaspoon lemon juice
1 tablespoon lemon zest
1 large egg

1/4 cup plain breadcrumbs
2 tablespoons mayo
1/4 cup grated Parmesan cheese
1 teaspoon dried parsley
4 tablespoons plain breadcrumbs
3 tablespoons grated Parmesan cheese
2 tablespoons olive oil divided

1. Start by draining canned tuna from water. I use a small colander to do that.
2. Next, combine it with garlic, onion, salt and pepper, lemon juice and zest, egg, breadcrumbs, mayo, 1/4 cup of grated Parmesan cheese and dried parsley. Mix well.

3. Combine remaining breadcrumbs and grated cheese in a shallow dish. Scoop 1/4 cup of tuna mixture, form into a patty and lightly coat with breading mixture.
4. Fry cake in pan with oil, until nicely browned on each side.
5. Remove from pan and let rest for 5 minutes.
6. Serve with spinach or other greens, additional lemon wedge or even simple aioli.

Tuna with Cheese and Three-Herb Pesto

Prep time: 25 minute | Cook time: 25 minute | Serves 4

1 lb fresh tuna steaks
1 teaspoon olive or vegetable oil
¼ teaspoon salt
1 cup loosely packed fresh cilantro leaves
½ cup loosely packed fresh flat-leaf parsley leaves
¼ cup loosely packed fresh basil leaves
4 medium green onions, sliced (1/4

cup)
1 clove garlic cut in half
2 tablespoons lime juice
2 teaspoons olive or vegetable oil
¼ teaspoon salt
¼ cup Progresso reduced-sodium chicken broth
1 tablespoon grated Parmesan cheese

1. Set oven control to broil. Brush both sides of tuna steaks with 1 teaspoon oil. Place on rack in broiler pan.
2. Broil with tops 4 inches from heat 8 to 10 minutes, turning once and sprinkling with 1/4 teaspoon salt, until tuna flakes easily with fork.
3. Meanwhile, in food processor bowl with metal blade, place remaining ingredients except broth and cheese. Cover and process about 10 seconds or until finely chopped.
4. With processor running, slowly pour in broth and continue processing until almost smooth. Stir in cheese. Serve with tuna.

Lime Sauce with Italian Crab Cakes

Prep time: 15 minute | Cook time: 20 minute | Serves 3

2 cans (6 ounces each) lump crabmeat, drained
1 green onion, chopped
1 tablespoon Dijon mustard
1 teaspoon Italian salad dressing mix
1-1/2 cups crushed butter-flavoured

crackers (about 35), divided
1 cup mayonnaise, divided
2 tablespoons lime juice, divided
1/4 cup canola oil
1/4 cup sour cream
1-1/2 teaspoons grated lime zest

1. In a large bowl, combine the crab, onion, and mustard, dressing mix, 1 cup cracker crumbs, 1/2 cup mayonnaise and 1 tablespoon lime juice.
2. Shape into six patties; coat with remaining cracker crumbs.
3. In a large skillet, heat oil over medium heat. Cook crab cakes for 3-4 minutes on each side or until lightly browned.
4. For lime sauce, in a small bowl, combine the sour cream, lime zest, and remaining mayonnaise and lime juice until blended. Serve with crab cakes.

Lemony Shrimp and Crabmeat Bowl

Prep time: 15 minute | Cook time: 20 minute | Serves 8

1 lb sourdough bread (455 g)
8 tablespoons unsalted butter
1 cup shredded cheddar cheese (100 g)
3 teaspoons kosher salt, divided
4 cups dry white wine (960 mL)
1 lb shrimp (455 g)
1 lb large scallops (455 g)
1 lb jumbo lump crabmeat (455 g)
2 cups half & half (480

mL)
3 tablespoons all-purpose flour
1 teaspoon Worcestershire sauce
1 teaspoon paprika
1 tablespoon lemon juice
2 tablespoons ketchup
28 oz artichoke heart (795 g), 2 cans, drained and chopped
Fresh chive, chopped, for garnish
Lemon wedge, for serving

1. Preheat the oven to 350°F (180°C).
2. Spread the bread in a single layer on a rimmed baking sheet and bake for 10 minutes, until lightly toasted. Let cool to room temperature. Leave the oven on.
3. Add the toasted bread to a food processor and pulse until finely ground.
4. In a large bowl, combine the bread crumbs, 4 tablespoons of melted butter, the cheddar cheese, and 1 teaspoon of salt and toss to combine. Set aside.
5. In a medium pot, combine 4 cups (960 ml) of white wine and a generous pinch of salt and bring to a boil over medium-high heat.
6. Add the shrimp and cook until bright pink, about 1 minute. Use a spider or slotted spoon to transfer the shrimp to a colander to drain.
7. Return the wine to a boil. Add the scallops and cook until just opaque, about 2 minutes. Transfer the scallops to a colander to drain.
8. Chop the shrimp and scallops into bite-size pieces.
9. Transfer to large bowl, along with the crab and 1 teaspoon of salt. Toss to combine.
10. In a liquid measuring cup or medium bowl, whisk together the half-and-half, 3 tablespoons of melted butter, the flour, Worcestershire sauce, paprika, lemon juice, ketchup, remaining tablespoon of white wine, and remaining teaspoon of salt.
11. Brush the remaining tablespoon of melted butter in a 9 x 13-inch (22 x 33 cm) baking dish.
12. Scatter the artichokes in an even layer over the bottom of the baking dish. Scoop the seafood mixture over the artichokes.
13. Pour the sauce over the seafood. Top with the bread crumb mixture.
14. Bake the casserole for 20-25 minutes, or until bubbling and golden brown.
15. Top with chives and serve with lemon wedges.

Mushroom & Shrimp with Snow Peas

Prep time: 10 minute | Cook time: 20 minute | Serves 4

2 tablespoons corn-starch
1 teaspoon sugar
1 teaspoon chicken bouillon granules
1 teaspoon dill weed
1/2 teaspoon salt
1/2 teaspoon grated lemon zest
1/8 teaspoon pepper
1 cup water
3 tablespoons lemon juice
1 pound uncooked medium shrimp,
peeled and deveined
2 cups sliced fresh mushrooms
1-1/2 cups sliced celery
1 medium sweet yellow or red pepper, julienned
1/4 cup thinly sliced green onions
1 tablespoon olive oil
6 ounces fresh or frozen snow peas, thawed
2 cups cooked rice

1. In a small bowl, combine the corn starch, sugar, bouillon, dill, salt, lemon zest and pepper. Stir in water and lemon juice until blended; set aside.
2. In a large nonstick skillet or wok, stir-fry the shrimp, mushrooms, celery, yellow pepper and onions in oil for 5 minutes.
3. Add the peas; stir-fry 1-2 minutes longer or until crisp-tender. Stir bouillon mixture; add to skillet.
4. Bring to a boil; cook and stir for 2 minutes or until thickened. Serve with rice.

Honey Garlic Paprika Salmon

Prep time: 10 minute | Cook time: 10 minute | Serves 4

3 Tablespoon butter
2 tsp olive oil
6 cloves garlic minced
1/2 cup honey
3 Tablespoon water
3 Tablespoon soy sauce
1 Tablespoon sriracha sauce
2 Tablespoon lemon
juice4 (6 oz each) salmon filets
1/2 tsp kosher salt
1/2 tsp black pepper
1/2 tsp smoked paprika (or regular paprika)
1/4 tsp blackening seasoning (optional)

1. Pat salmon dry, then season with salt, pepper, paprika and blackening seasoning (if using). Set aside. Adjust oven rack to middle position, then preheat broiler.

2. Add butter and oil to a large, oven-safe skillet over high heat. Once hi is melted, add garlic, water, soy sauce, sriracha, honey and lemon juice and cook 30 seconds or so, until sauce is heated through.
3. Add salmon, skin side down (if using salmon with skin), and cook 3 minutes. While salmon cooks, baste frequently with sauce from the pan by spooning it over the top of the salmon.
4. Broil salmon for 5-6 minutes, basting with sauce once during the broil, until salmon is caramelized and cooked to desired doneness.
5. Garnish with minced parsley if desired.

Low Fat Buttery Oyster Stew

Prep time: 15 minute | Cook time: 30 minute | Serves 6

3 tablespoons butter
2 cups diced white onion
1 cup diced celery, plus 1/4 cup chopped celery leaves, divided
2 pints shucked oysters, liquid reserved
¾ teaspoon kosher
salt
½ teaspoon paprika
3 ½ cups low-fat milk
½ cup heavy cream
3 dashes hot sauce
Freshly ground pepper to taste
2 tablespoons snipped fresh chives

1. Heat butter in a large saucepan over medium heat until melted. Add onion and diced celery; reduce heat to medium-low and cook, stirring occasionally, until translucent and very tender but not browned, 25 to 30 minutes.
2. Meanwhile, cut oysters in half or quarters, depending on size. Pour the oyster liquid through a fine-mesh sieve to strain out any grit.
3. Stir salt and paprika into the vegetables and cook, stirring, for 1 minute more. Add the strained oyster liquid, milk, cream and hot sauce. Increase heat to high and bring to a boil
4. Reduce heat to a simmer and gently add the oysters. Cook just until their edges begin to curl, 2 to 3 minute.
5. Remove from heat. Season with pepper. Garnish with celery leaves and chives.

Coconut Salmon with Scallion Greens

Prep time: 10 minute | Cook time: 15 minutes | Serves 2

2 (6-ounce) salmon fillets
¼ cup white or yellow miso
2 tablespoons rice or coconut vinegar
2 tablespoons sesame oil, divided
1 tablespoon gluten-free soy sauce, tamari, or coconut amino
1 tablespoon minced fresh ginger
1 clove garlic, minced
1½ pounds (medium bunch) baby bok choy, core removed, sliced into 1½-inch pieces, white stem and leafy green parts separated
2 tablespoons thinly sliced scallion whites (optional)
2 tablespoons thinly sliced scallion greens, for garnish (optional)

1. Heat the broiler to high.
2. On a baking sheet or broiler pan, place the salmon, skin-side down, and pat it dry.
3. In a small bowl, whisk together the miso, vinegar, 1 tablespoon of the sesame oil, the soy sauce, ginger, and garlic.
4. Spread 2 tablespoons of the glaze evenly over the top of the salmon, setting aside the remainder. Let it stand for 10 minutes, if you have time.
5. Broil the salmon until the glaze is bubbly, 3 to 4 minutes.
6. Cover it loosely with foil and continue to broil until slightly pink in the center, another 3 to 4 minutes.
7. Remove the salmon from the broiler, remove the foil, and let it cool.
8. In a large skillet over medium-high heat, heat the remaining 1 tablespoon sesame oil.
9. Add the bok choy stems and scallion whites (if using) and cook until just tender, 2 to 3 minutes.
10. Stir in the remaining miso glaze and cook until fragrant, 30 to 60 seconds.
11. Add the bok choy greens, cover, and steam until just wilted, 30 seconds. Toss to coat with the sauce.
12. To serve, divide the bok choy evenly between two plates. Top each with a salmon fillet and sprinkle with scallion greens (if using).

Soy dipped Avocado Sushi Roll

Prep time: 15 minute | Cook time: 0 minute | Serves 2

2 sheets sushi nori
1 medium avocado, pitted and peeled
2 tablespoons sesame seeds, divided (optional)
4 ounces smoked salmon (about 4 thin slices)
1 medium cucumber,
cut into matchsticks
3 tablespoons pickled ginger (optional)
1 teaspoon wasabi paste (optional)
Gluten-free soy sauce, tamari, or coconut amino, for dipping

1. Lay 1 piece of nori on a sheet of parchment paper or aluminium foil on a flat surface.
2. In a small bowl, mash the avocado with a fork.
3. Spread half of the avocado mixture on the nori sheet, leaving a ½-inch strip uncovered along the top edge.
4. Sprinkle 1 tablespoon of the sesame seeds (if using), evenly over the avocado. Arrange 2 pieces of the smoked salmon horizontally, covering the avocado.
5. Arrange the cucumber horizontally, running up the length of the sheet and creating columns to cover the salmon.
6. Wet the tip of your finger and run it along the exposed seam. Roll the nori tightly away from you, using the foil as a guide and pressing firmly to seal.
7. Repeat the process with the remaining nori sheet and ingredients, and refrigerate both for at least 30 minutes to firm up.
8. Using a very sharp or serrated knife, slice each roll into 6 to 8 pieces. Serve with pickled ginger and wasabi and soy sauce for dipping

Spicy Cilantro Fish wrapped in Lettuce Leaves

Prep time: 30 minute | Cook time: 20 minute | Serves 4

1¼ pounds meaty skinless fresh fish fillets (wild-caught or Hamachi tuna, halibut, tilapia, barramundi, or mahi mahi), cut into ½-inch cubes
3 tablespoons lime juice
3 tablespoons lemon juice
¼ teaspoon salt
¼ teaspoons freshly ground black pepper
2 ripe plum or heirloom tomatoes, seeded and chopped (juices reserved)
1 tablespoon olive oil
¾ cup chopped red onion
1 Serrano pepper, seeded and minced (optional)
Bibb lettuce leaves, for serving
4 avocados
Juice from ½ lime (reserve remaining half for wedges, for serving)
½ cup chopped fresh cilantro
2 tablespoons chopped red onion
1 Serrano pepper, seeded and minced
Chopped fresh cilantro
Lime wedges

1. In a medium bowl, place the fish, lime and lemon juices, salt, and pepper and toss to combine.
2. Cover tightly and chill until the fish turns completely white, tossing occasionally, at least 4 hours and up to 6 hours.
3. Meanwhile, make the guacamole. Cut the avocados in half, and then remove the pit and peel.
4. Spoon the avocado into a large bowl and mash it with a large metal spoon.
5. Add the lime juice and continue to mix and mash until mostly smooth with some remaining chunks (this helps prevent the guacamole from browning).
6. Mix in the cilantro, onion, and Serrano pepper. Cover tightly and refrigerate until ready to use.
7. Strain the fish, moving it to a clean bowl; discard the marinade. Add the tomatoes, oil, onion, and Serrano pepper (if using) and toss gently to combine.
8. Serve wrapped in the lettuce leaves topped with the guacamole and your choice of additional fixings.

Homemade Shrimp and Pea Bowl with Cashews

Prep time: 15 minute | Cook time: 20 minute | Serves 4

3 tablespoons gluten-free soy sauce, tamari, or coconut amino
2 tablespoons minced fresh ginger
3 tablespoons sesame oil, divided
2 large eggs, lightly beaten
⅔ to ¾ pound medium shrimp, peeled and deveined (about 24)
1 shallot, minced
1 red bell pepper, seeded and diced
¾ cup frozen peas
¼ cup chopped unsalted cashews
2 tablespoons chopped fresh cilantro
¼ teaspoon red pepper flakes (optional)
Sliced scallion greens, for garnish (optional)

1. In a small bowl, whisk the soy sauce and ginger together and set aside.
2. In a wok or large skillet over medium heat, heat 1 tablespoon of the sesame oil.
3. Add the eggs and cook, stirring frequently with a wooden spoon or spatula, until scrambled.
4. Transfer to a small bowl and break up the cooked egg into small pieces using two forks. Set aside.
5. In the same wok over medium-high heat, heat 1 tablespoon of the sesame oil.
6. Add the shrimp and cook, tossing, until bright pink but not browned, 3 to 4 minutes.
7. Transfer the shrimp to a separate plate or bowl and set aside.
8. Add the remaining 1 tablespoon sesame oil and the shallot to the wok and cook until fragrant, tossing frequently, about 30 seconds.
9. Add the bell pepper and cook until just tender, tossing occasionally, about 2 minutes.
10. Add the cauliflower rice and cook, tossing occasionally, until lightly browned and crisp, about 5 minutes.
11. Stir in the soy sauce mixture. Add the cooked shrimp, cooked eggs, and peas and stir until well combined and heated through, 2 to 3 minutes.
12. Add the cashews, cilantro, and red pepper flakes (if using), tossing to combine.
13. Divide the mixture among four bowls, garnish with scallion greens (if using) and serve.

Mussel Spinach Cold Butter Bowl

Prep time: 10 minute | Cook time: 8 minute | Serves 4

2 pounds mussels
1 tablespoon extra-virgin olive oil
2 shallots, minced
3 cloves garlic, minced
¼ cup lemon juice (from 2 lemons)
¼ cup chopped fresh parsley, plus more for garnish
¼ cup chopped fresh dill (optional)
3 tablespoons

chopped fresh thyme
½ teaspoon salt
¼ teaspoons freshly ground black pepper
¼ teaspoon red pepper flakes (optional)
3 cups baby spinach (or spinach leaves torn into smaller pieces)
2 tablespoons cold unsalted grass-fed butter, cubed

1. Rinse the mussels under cold running water, pulling off their black beards as needed. Place in a strainer to drain and set aside.
2. Heat the oil in a large, deep skillet, stockpot, or Dutch oven over medium-high heat.
3. Add the shallots and cook, stirring, until soft and translucent, about 2 minutes.
4. Add the garlic and cook until fragrant, 30 seconds. Add the stock, lemon juice, herbs, salt, pepper, and red pepper flakes (if using), and stirring to combine. Bring the stock to a boil.
5. Add the mussels, cover, and cook, undisturbed, until the mussels open their shells, about 5 minutes.
6. Reduce the heat to low. Discard any mussels that have not yet opened. Divide the mussels among four large serving bowls.
7. Add the spinach to the broth, cover, and cook until just wilted, 1 to 2 minutes. Remove the lid and turn off the heat. Let sit for 1 minute, then add the cold butter, one piece at a time, stirring in each one until fully melted before adding the next one.
8. Spoon the broth over the mussels in the bowls, garnish with more parsley if you like, and serve.

My Special Pepper Shrimp with Spinach

Prep time: 10 minute | Cook time: 10 minute | Serves 4

3 tablespoons extra-virgin olive oil, divided
6 cloves garlic, minced
1 cup unsalted chicken broth or stock
Grated zest and juice from 1 medium lemon
½ teaspoon red pepper flakes, or to taste
¼ teaspoon sea salt or Himalayan salt, or

to taste
½ teaspoon freshly ground black pepper, or to taste
¼ cup (½ stick) cold unsalted grass-fed butter, cubed
6 to 8 cups (6 ounces) baby spinach leaves
2 to 3 tablespoons chopped fresh parsley (optional)

1. Pat the shrimp very dry with paper towels. Heat 2 tablespoons of the olive oil in a large skillet over medium-high heat.
2. Add the shrimp and cook until pink, flipping once, about 2 minutes per side. Transfer to a large bowl or plate.
3. Reduce the heat to medium and add remaining 1 tablespoon oil. Add the garlic and cook until just fragrant, about 1 minute.
4. Add the broth, lemon zest and juice, red pepper flakes, salt, and black pepper, increase the heat to medium-high, and bring to a simmer.
5. Reduce the sauce by half, scraping up any browned bits from the bottom with a wooden spoon, about 5 minutes.
6. Remove the pan from the heat and allow cooling slightly. Add butter, one cube at a time, stirring continually with a wooden spoon until the sauce thickens.
7. To serve, divide spinach evenly among four plates.
8. Top each plate with about 4 shrimp. Divide the sauce evenly among the plates and garnish with the parsley (if using).

APPENDIX 1 MEASUREMENT CONVERSION CHART

VOLUME EQUIVALENTS(DRY)

US STANDARD	METRIC (APPROXIMATE)
1/8 teaspoon	0.5 mL
1/4 teaspoon	1 mL
1/2 teaspoon	2 mL
3/4 teaspoon	4 mL
1 teaspoon	5 mL
1 tablespoon	15 mL
1/4 cup	59 mL
1/2 cup	118 mL
3/4 cup	177 mL
1 cup	235 mL
2 cups	475 mL
3 cups	700 mL
4 cups	1 L

VOLUME EQUIVALENTS(LIQUID)

US STANDARD	US STANDARD (OUNCES)	METRIC (APPROXIMATE)
2 tablespoons	1 fl.oz.	30 mL
1/4 cup	2 fl.oz.	60 mL
1/2 cup	4 fl.oz.	120 mL
1 cup	8 fl.oz.	240 mL
1 1/2 cup	12 fl.oz.	355 mL
2 cups or 1 pint	16 fl.oz.	475 mL
4 cups or 1 quart	32 fl.oz.	1 L
1 gallon	128 fl.oz.	4 L

TEMPERATURES EQUIVALENTS

FAHRENHEIT(F)	CELSIUS(C) (APPROXIMATE)
225 °F	107 °C
250 °F	120 °C
275 °F	135 °C
300 °F	150 °C
325 °F	160 °C
350 °F	180 °C
375 °F	190 °C
400 °F	205 °C
425 °F	220 °C
450 °F	235 °C
475 °F	245 °C
500 °F	260 °C

WEIGHT EQUIVALENTS

US STANDARD	METRIC (APPROXIMATE)
1 ounce	28 g
2 ounces	57 g
5 ounces	142 g
10 ounces	284 g
15 ounces	425 g
16 ounces (1 pound)	455 g
1.5 pounds	680 g
2 pounds	907 g

APPENDIX 2 THE DIRTY DOZEN AND CLEAN FIFTEEN

The Environmental Working Group (EWG) is a nonprofit, nonpartisan organization dedicated to protecting human health and the environment Its mission is to empower people to live healthier lives in a healthier environment. This organization publishes an annual list of the twelve kinds of produce, in sequence, that have the highest amount of pesticide residue-the Dirty Dozen-as well as a list of the fifteen kinds ofproduce that have the least amount of pesticide residue-the Clean Fifteen.

THE DIRTY DOZEN

- The 2016 Dirty Dozen includes the following produce. These are considered among the year's most important produce to buy organic:

Strawberries	Spinach
Apples	Tomatoes
Nectarines	Bell peppers
Peaches	Cherry tomatoes
Celery	Cucumbers
Grapes	Kale/collard greens
Cherries	Hot peppers

- The Dirty Dozen list contains two additional itemskale/collard greens and hot peppers-because they tend to contain trace levels of highly hazardous pesticides.

THE CLEAN FIFTEEN

- The least critical to buy organically are the Clean Fifteen list. The following are on the 2016 list:

Avocados	Papayas
Corn	Kiw
Pineapples	Eggplant
Cabbage	Honeydew
Sweet peas	Grapefruit
Onions	Cantaloupe
Asparagus	Cauliflower
Mangos	

- Some of the sweet corn sold in the United States are made from genetically engineered (GE) seedstock. Buy organic varieties of these crops to avoid GE produce.

APPENDIX 3 RECIPE INDEX

Homemade Tomato Cilantro Sauce 124
Homemade Turkey Cranberry Salad with Kiwi 51
Homemade Vanilla Hot Cereal 73
Homemade White pepper Tomato Pasta 63
Homemade zucchini Carrot Smoothie 66
Homemade-Coconut Oil Baked Seeds Mix 86
Honey Garlic Paprika Salmon 155
Hot & Spicy Pineapple Coconut Chicken 55
Hot and Spicy Garlic Broccoli with Bell Peppers 112
Hot and Spicy Onion Ground Cumin Sauce 128
Hot and Spicy Yellow Pepper-Potato Puree 132
Hot and Spicy Zucchini Sticks 80
Hot Sweet Potato Vegetable Pasta 62
Indian spiced Crispy Kale Chips 82
Instant Cantaloupe Blueberry Salad 103
Instant Moist Eggs with scallion greens 29
Instant Parmesan Halibut 58
Instant Pepper Shrimp Snap Pea Curry 151
Instant Quinoa and Black Bean Salad 37
Instant Spicy Cucumber Onion Salad 100
Instant Tasty Cheesy Pizza with Tomato sauce 39

J-K
Juicy Tomato Grass-fed Beef with Pepper 137
Kale and Golden Beets Peppery Salad 108
Kale Pesto Almond Soup 106
Lemony Avocado Salman Wraps 22
Lemony Basil Tomato Vegetable Soup 40

L
Lemony Coconut Mango Bowl 96
Lemony Dates with Hazelnuts 88
Lemony Garlic Broccoli with Hazelnuts 116
Lemony Grapefruit Watercress Smoothie 66
Lemony Lettuce Bell pepper Salad with Fennel 44
Lemony Quinoa Salad with Peppery Tuna 31
Lemony Radish Chickpea Salad 42
Lemony Raspberry Sauce 123
Lemony Shredded Cabbage Salad 115
Lemony Shrimp & Bell pepper Salad 44
Lemony Shrimp and Crabmeat Bowl 154
Lemony Sole Fry with Chopped Scallions 53
Lemony Tarragon Salad dressing 106
Lettuce & Double Berry Smoothie 67
Lime Sauce with Italian Crab Cakes 154
Low Fat Buttery Oyster Stew 155
Low Sodium Turnip Salad   113

Macadamia Snack with Egg fills and Raspberry Sauce 90

M-N
Magic Cauliflower Leek Sauce 127
Magic Garlic Onion Artichoke Sauce 131
Magical Dried Fruit and Nut curry 83
Mango Tangerines and Cilantro Bowl 80
Maple based Walnut and Beets with Goat Cheese 114
Maple Fig Jam 125
Maple Pineapple with Macadamia Nuts 92
Maple Walnut Almond Granola 22
Marinated Steak Skewers with Chimichurri Sauce 61
Milky Watermelon Salad 102
Mom's Special Blueberry Coconut Muffins 93
Muenster -Bacon Stuffed Chicken Breast 52
Mulberry-Pistachio Salad 86
Mushroom & Shrimp with Snow Peas 155
Mushroom and Vegetables with Pepper 83
Mushroom Coconut Cream Soup 39
Mushroom Thyme and Celery Soup 106
Mushroom- Bacon Egg fills 19
Mussel Spinach Cold Butter Bowl 158
My Special Pepper Shrimp with Spinach 158
Natural Vanilla Avocado Smoothie 69
No sugar Orange Juice Apple Pie 92
Nutty Fruity Chicken Zucchini Noodles 56
Nutty Fruity Pies 92

O
Olive Oil Roasted Almonds 83
One pan Broiled Salmon with Yellow Miso 144
One Pan Mushroom with Sautéed Almonds 111
One Pan Pork Lion with Brussels 134
One Pan Pork with apple-onion relish 138
One Pan Rainbow Butter Trout with Lemon 148
One pan Roasted vegetables with jalapeño peppers 115
One pot Chicken with Guar Parsley and Sauce 60
One Pot Mustard Chicken with Bacon and Onions 50
Onion Black pepper Corn Salad 112
Onion Coconut milk Chicken with almonds 141
Orange & Tomato based Fennel 119
Oven Baked Asparagus with Eggs and Tomatoes 23

Oven cooked Chicken with bacon Asiago cheese 52

P

Paleo Baby Greens & Raspberries Goat Cheese Salad 101

Paleo Cauliflower Gnocchi with spinach 32

Paleo Chicken Pomegranate Salad 141

Paleo Lean Beef Vegetables Soup 142

Peaches Crisp with Almond and coconut flakes 26

Pecan and Walnut Holiday Nut Mix 87

Pegan Chicken Onion and Carrot Soup 140

Pegan Grilled Soy Steak and Baby Spinach 136

Pepper Roasted Squash 110

Peppery Balsamic Marinade   104

Peppery Beef Roast with gravy 53

Peppery Cauliflower Beets Salad 46

Peppery Egg with Italian Bread 27

Peppery Eggs with Lemon Hollandaise Sauce 28

Peppery Lettuce Chicken Roll 19

Peppery Shrimp and Steak for Two 143

Peppery Sweet Potato and Scrambled Eggs 20

Perfect Broccoli scrambled eggs 36

Perfectly Roasted Parsnip Chips 86

Poached Apple and Pears with Cinnamon 25

Protein rich Garlic Edamame Dip 128

Q-R

Quick & Fresh Thyme Tomato Sauce 128

Quick Ginger-Garlic Miso Dressing 128

Quinoa and Cinnamon Butternut Squash Salad 113

Quinoa with Peppery Oyster Mushrooms 61

Raisin Walnut Cookies 91

Restaurant style Spicy Salsa 81

Rice Milk Blueberry Muffins 26

Rich Garlic Soy Sauce 130

Rich Garlic Thyme Mushroom Stock 104

Roasted Apples Brussels Mix 112

Roasted Carrot Parsnips & Sweet Potato Bowl 113

Rosemary Green Beans Millet Salad 46

Rosemary Pepper Chicken with Broccoli Florets 49

Rutabaga Turnip Vegetable Salad 42

S

Salmon Avocado Coconut Milk Soup 149

Salmon Egg Sandwich with Avocado 29

Salty Brown Apple 88

Scallion Mushroom Zoodles Salad with Basil 33

Scallion parsley Egg Omelet 27

Scallions and Oyster Mushroom Sauce 132

Scrambled Pepper Egg 119

Seasonal Vegetable Mix 112

Shallot & Wild Rice with Mushroom Soup 40

Shrimp Coconut Chicken Soup 148

Shrimp Cucumber Noodles with Chili Sauce 150

Shrimp Lettuce Garden Salad 147

Simple and Easy Tender Lemony Artichokes 109

Simple Belgian endive Egg with Cheese and Onion   31

Simple Lemon Garlic Shrimp Bowl 151

Simple Raw Tomato Juice 77

Simple Vegan Brownies 78

Six Ingredients- Feel Fresh Smoothie 68

Soy dipped Avocado Sushi Roll 156

Spaghetti Squash Beef with Black Pepper and Basil 137

Spiced Trout with Smoky seasoning   30

Spicy Apple Pears Jam 127

Spicy Beef and Tomato Coconut Curry 120

Spicy Carrot Root Soup 43

Spicy Chicken with Fresh Cilantro 49

Spicy Cilantro Fish wrapped in Lettuce Leaves 157

Spicy Coconut Sweet Potato with Kale 32

Spicy Crabs with Chilled Coleslaw Mix 145

Spicy Egg pepper Zoodles with Avocado 18

Spicy Eggplant Tahini Spread 124

Spicy Garlic Roasted Almonds 85

Spicy Garlicky Tomato Onion Omelet 30

Spicy Ground Chicken with Lime and Soy Sauce140

Spicy Onion Collard Greens Mix 111

Spicy Parsley Cilantro Sauce 126

Spicy Pasta with Mackerel and Breadcrumbs 39

Spicy Peppery Chicken Lettuce Wraps 135

Spicy Peppery Green Beans with Baby Peas 110

Spicy Rice milk Egg Muffins 27

Spicy Tasty Tahini Date & Carrot Salad 42

Spicy Turkey and vegetables Soup 51

Spicy Vegan Paprika Garlic Cashew Cream 129

Spinach and Berry with Chicken Salad 139

Spinach Avocado Salad with Watermelon 41

Spinach Tomato Blast Smoothie 69

Spinach Zucchini Green Smoothie   66

Spinach Zucchini Smoothie 71

CPSIA information can be obtained
at www.ICGtesting.com
Printed in the USA
BVHW091049091221
623631BV00003B/242